# TEXTBOOK OF
# OCCUPATIONAL THERAPY

# TEXTBOOK OF
# OCCUPATIONAL THERAPY

### With Chief Reference To Psychological Medicine

EAMON N. M. O'SULLIVAN

B.A., M.B., D.P.M.

LONDON

H. K. LEWIS & Co. Ltd.

1955

*Printed in the Republic of Ireland by*
THE KERRYMAN LTD., TRALEE

# CONTENTS

v

# FOREWORD

HAVING BEEN PRIVILEGED to read the manuscript on occupational therapy by Eamon N. M. O'Sullivan, M.B., it seems proper to express my opinion of this work.

It is pleasant to be able to say that I know of no other work on the subject, hitherto seen, which is so complete and specific. One cannot fail to admire the diligence of the author in his research and in the use of the material he has gathered. His conclusions appear to be most orthodox and in keeping with the opinion expressed by other writers on occupational therapy.

These are presented in a clear, most readable style which makes perusal of the work a pleasure rather than a task. There is never doubt in the reader's mind that the author is expressing his opinions in a manner that permits no mis-interpretation of them.

Dr. O'Sullivan has admirably epitomised the subject of mental disorders and given hints for occupational treatment of such patients, but throughout the book emphasises the importance of consideration of the individual in prescribing occupational therapy for mental patients.

While the author has written primarily for those who are connected with mental hospitals, there are numerous refer-ences to general, surgical, orthopaedic and other special hospitals. Therefore, there is much in the book which will be informative and stimulating to all who are interested in occupational therapy.

The book should be of value to administrative officers who are contemplating the inauguration of an occupational therapy department under their charge, but those who have been familiar with, or have been prescribing or practising occupational therapy for a number of years, will gain much inspiration and knowledge from its pages.

The chapters on the organization of a department of occupational therapy in a large mental hospital are admirable in their specificity and should prove of great assistance to those to whom such a duty might fall, but there is one warning must be given the reader in order to emphasize what the author has already said. In detailing the requirements for equipment and materials, lists are given which are utopian in scope. While the author states that such plans must be gradually put in operation I feel this should be emphasized more emphatically.

I have pleasure in recommending the Text to all those interested in or concerned with the development of occupational therapy.

William Rush Dunton.

# CHAPTER I.

## INTRODUCTION

THE IMPORTANCE OF occupational therapy has been recognised over the centuries, since the time of Galen's famous second century dictum—'Employment is nature's best physician, and is essential to human happiness.'

It, however, received its greatest impetus, following the two recent world wars. Medical acknowledgement of its value, for treatment purposes, became fairly universal in the last century, but it is in the present century, particularly following the 1914-'18 war, that the development of its curative properties became established on scientific lines. The mental and physical rehabilitation of the war casualties, then increasing in fairly large numbers, called for the rapid organisation of suitable occupational therapy services. The success attending these services has stimulated increased recognition, both medical and lay, in the therapeutic and rehabilitative nature of O.T. So, to-day, this branch of medical science has developed into a fully-fledged and acknowledged speciality in most countries.

Because of its infancy in development, there is a dearth of suitable texts, dealing exclusively with the subject. There is, particularly, a necessity for textbooks, sufficiently comprehensive and detailed, to meet the teaching needs in the new and expanding profession associated with O.T. There is now a general demand for a textbook, compiled in the closest possible conformity with the current teaching syllabus of the courses laid down for the training of occupational therapists. These training syllabuses are, in general, somewhat similar in Great Britain, Canada and U.S.A., and these countries are in the forefront in the scientific organisation and expansion of occupational therapy in all its many phases.

The author, mindful of shortcomings and other defects, which are a human inherency, has humbly attempted to do an individual's part, in compiling such a textbook, which, is hoped, should prove a sincere effort to approach these requirements. It is offered, too, following almost a life study of the subject, as a contribution to stimulate further interest in a science which has tremendous possibilities in the re-habilitation of the mentally and physically ill and which, quite often, is the only sheet-anchor of importance in the treatment and handling of the chronic grades in both types.

For obvious reasons, the text, herewith, deals mainly with the psychological application of the treatment, though its value in the case of physical ailments, both surgical and medical, is not under-stressed throughout the work. It is not possible to deal comprehensively with both aspects in one textbook. In fact, a few practical treatises, even if limited in scope, covering the occupational treatment of physical diseases and mainly concerning surgical conditions, have been published in recent years. This differentiation has become an unavoidable necessity, just as in the case of texts on medicine and surgery and even other medical specialties.

In conclusion, I am glad to acknowledge my indebtedness to Dr. W. R. Dunton, Jr., of Catonsville, Maryland, U.S.A., for his valuable advice and assistance and his kindness in reading over the draft of the entire text and writing such an encouraging foreword. Dr. Dunton is the recognised leading American authority on occupational therapy. He has performed monumental work in the founding of the *American Journal of Occupational Therapy* and in acting as its first Editor for a lengthy period. He was also actively associated with the establishment and subsequent develop-ment of the American Association of Occupational Therapists.

I am also indebted to a number of friends, who kindly assisted in typing the material, but I owe my chief inspiration to the encouragement received from my wife and family— *Forsan et haec olim meminisse juvabit.*—Virgil.

Eamon N. M. O'Sullivan.

Mental Hospital, Killarney,
March, 1955.

## CHAPTER II.

## DEFINITION AND HISTORY

OCCUPATIONAL THERAPY, as the term itself conveys, is merely treatment by means of suitable occupation—the word 'Therapy' being derived from the Greek word 'Therapeia' which means curing or medical treatment. It will be noted that the word 'Therapy' occupies the position of maximum importance in the title and is merely qualified by the word 'Occupational' to indicate the type of treatment. This distinguishes it immediately from the use of occupations for any purpose other than therapeutic. In many mental hospitals, especially prior to the 1914-'18 War, occupations were considered more from the economic than the curative aspect. Patients were detailed for work in the Farm, Garden, Kitchen, Laundry, Tradesmen's Shops, etc., often with the emphasis on reducing hospital costs and sometimes without due regard for the prognosis in each individual case.

The term *Ergotherapy* has also been used, which simply means 'work' therapy, but the restrictive nature of this title, which does not embrace any reference to many occupational activities, apart from work proper, such as recreations, hobbies, etc., renders it unacceptable and the more suitable term 'occupational therapy' is now universally approved. The term *Diversional Therapy* has also been used, but is not sufficiently explicit and merely characterises one of the main sections of occupational therapy.

Various definitions of occupational therapy have been given, some of a most comprehensive nature and exceeding all the canons laid down for a logical definition, but, as they are descriptive and most informative, some of them are quoted. The Walter Reed General Hospital, Washington, U.S.A., gives the following:—

'Occupational Therapy is a term now applied to that form of remedial treatment consisting of various forms of activity, mental or physical, which relieve a patient temporarily, or which either

I

contribute to or hasten recovery from disease or injury. This activity under medical supervision or guidance is consciously motivated.'

The Board of Control in England, in its memorandum of 1933, has the following definition:—

'Occupational Therapy is the treatment, under medical direction, of physical or mental disorders by the application of occupation and recreation, with the object of promoting recovery, of creating new habits and of preventing deterioration.'

The United States Veterans' Administration has elaborated the following:—

'Occupational Therapy is that form of treatment, which includes any occupation, mental or physical, definitely prescribed and guided for the distinct purpose of contributing to and hastening recovery from disease or injury and of assisting in the social and institutional adjustment of individuals requiring long and indefinite periods of hospitalisation.'

The following very elaborate and comprehensive definition has been issued by the Boston School of Occupational Therapy, U.S.A.:—

'Occupational Therapy aims to furnish a scheme of scientifically arranged activities, which will give, to any set of muscles or related parts of the body in cases of disease or injury, just the degree of movement and exercise that may be directed by a competent physician or surgeon. Stimulating heart action, respiration and blood circulation accurately, as prescribed, and at the same time, it yields some of the joy and satisfaction that wisely selected, wholesome occupation provides in normal life. It thus takes its place with nursing, medicine and surgery as one of the important departments of medical art.'

Various other definitions have appeared from time to time, mostly of a descriptive type, but none sufficiently logical to justify being termed 'a definition.' The following definition should meet the case:—

Occupational Therapy is the treatment, under expert medical supervision, of mental or physical disease, by means of suitable occupation, whether mental, physical, social or recreational.

This definition shows that occupational therapy is a form of therapeusis or treatment differing from all other forms of treatment in its applicability to both mental and physical disease by means of occupation, whether the occupation be mental or physical, social or recreational, provided always that it be suitable and definitely prescribed by competent medical supervisors. The word 'suitable' has been introduced into the definition with regard to the occupation prescribed, to indicate that every form of occupation, though classed as such, may not be therapeutically desirable. Individual cases require individual attention and what may have curative results in one case or group of cases, may have vastly different results in others. Hence, in the prescription of suitable occupation, many considerations, psychological, physiological, orthopaedic, etc., may enter into the picture.

Psychiatrists, Physicians and Surgeons associated with occupational therapy in their different spheres, must have a sound and expert knowledge of the principles of occupational therapy. It is not sufficient to have nominal medical supervision. The medical director must be conversant with the theory and, to some extent, the practice of the treatment. It will be noted, too, that the treatment is applicable to both mental and physical disease and this is made clear in all the definitions given. While its use, as an adjunct to the treatment of all forms of mental disease, is now fairly universal in most countries, it has also been adapted for bodily ailments and physical disabilities. Medical Directors of Tubercular Sanatoria have for long appreciated its advantages as a practical form of treatment in suitable cases. Its recognition in the field of orthopaedics has become widespread and is proving most beneficial in conjunction with physiotherapy and other methods of treatment. It is also building up a reputation for itself in general hospitals in many countries. Here, again, it is co-related with the physiotherapy and other departments and availed of in many cardiac and other suitable cases. As a potent factor in convalescence from all ailments, it has become an important item in the treatment of such cases, especially those of the prolonged type, where the difficulties of planning a satisfactory daily time-table, otherwise, must constitute a tremendous deterrent against recovery.

Also, the definition, in addition to describing the occupation to be prescribed as suitable, qualifies it further as mental or physical. This is inserted to embrace all forms of treatment, from the purely physical occupation, ranging through the recreational to the social type, such as physical drill, dancing, music, social clubs and libraries, visits, hobbies, games, etc. It must be appreciated that the patient, who looks forward with obvious interest to the perusal of his daily newspaper, is as active a recipient of occupational therapy as the patient who passes from the rand to the wale in the completion of a basket. It is this diversity in the application of the treatment that constitutes the novelty, glamour and success of the therapy, which will be amplified in later chapters.

### History of Occupational Therapy

In reviewing the history of the use of occupations for curative purposes, it is impossible to say when and where occupations and handicrafts were first utilised as a definite form of treatment. From the very earliest times, it was realised that occupation, whether of necessity or as a hobby, promoted health and well-being and work was suggested as an antidote to worry and depression. Just as rational methods in medicine date from the time of the famous Hippocrates, the Father of Medicine, (460-370 B.C.), it is not surprising that the first authentic reference to the utility of occupation as a curative agent should emanate from another famous Greek physician, Galen, who is reputed to have said, sometime about the year 170 A.D., that 'Employment is nature's best physician and is essential to human happiness.' Many similar references were made in succeeding years. Philippe Pinel, about 1790 and his successor, Esquirol who, with William Tuke in England about the same period, sponsored the adoption of more humane methods of treatment for the mentally ill, also advocated the use of occupations as a form of treatment. Esquirol described work as:

'A stimulant to all, for by it we distract attention from their illness, we fix their attention on reasonable things; we bring back to them some of the practices of order; we quicken their intelligence and, in this way, we improve the lot of the most unfortunate.'

About the same period in Germany, Johann Freiderick Reil wrote a book on insanity, dealing at length with work as a curative agent. In it he described work as 'an excellent means to cure insanity. It must be wholesome and, whenever possible, be done in the open air and combined with exercise and change.'

About the same period, a little over a century ago in America, Eddy, Arnold and Rush were similarly disposed. The former made special recommendations for treating the insane on occupational lines in New York. Samuel Tuke, of The Retreat, York, England, is reported to have written to Eddy, as follows:—

'I observe with pleasure that one of the leading features of your new institution is the introduction of employment among the patients, an object which I am persuaded is of the utmost importance in the moral treatment of insanity. It is related of an Institution in Spain, which accommodated all ranks and in which the lower class were generally employed, that a greater proportion of these recovered, while the number of the grandees was exceedingly small.'

In 1846, Dr. John M. Galt, Medical Superintendent of the Eastern Lunatic Asylum, Williamsburg, Virginia, U.S.A., wrote:—

'No class of patients is so happy as the labourers; no other convalescents recover so rapidly and favourably; many of these would be completely miserable without labour and their recovery retarded. The patient enters by it into accustomed channels of thought and action, and the mind performs rationally at labour, if insane everywhere else. We think highly of employment to procure rest, give strength, promote appetite and facilitate recovery. When our patients begin to mend, they desire employment. Common amusements of Hospitals are useful and far better than nothing, but will not compare with labour as a means of restoration. It is true that "all work and no play makes Jack a dull boy." It is no less true, that all play and no work becomes insipid after a while and does not give that healthy impulse to the mind which the idea of utility in labour is sure to impart.'

Mention should be made here that, prior to the eighteenth century, sufferers from mental disease were treated as outcasts. Insanity was regarded as a punishment—a visitation from God. Those affected were deemed the victims of demoniacal possession and exorcism was rampant as the sole form of treatment. No special provision was made for proper segregation and, generally, those unmanageable were confined to prisons, chained and manacled, and often cruelly and barbarously treated. This was the degraded position of the insane, which Pinel in France, Reil in Germany, William Tuke in England, devoted most of their time to reform. The chains and manacles were dispensed with and special institutions for the insane were established, until recently, known as 'asylums.' They are now correctly designated as mental hospitals.

William Tuke, in 1792, founded the first in England, known as The Retreat near York and it is still so named. A book, written in 1813, by Samuel Tuke, a grandson of the founder, entitled a *Description of the Retreat*, expounded the principles of treatment adopted in this York Hospital, giving due prominence to the curative side of occupations. A writer in the *Edinburgh Review* at the time, commenting on the success of Tuke's experiment, stated:—

> 'An example has been set of courage, patience and kindness, which cannot be too highly commended, or too widely diffused and which will gradually bring into repute a milder and better method of treating the insane.'

It is noteworthy that, with the introduction of such humane reforms in all countries, work and occupation were mentioned prominently as therapeutic aids.

Although from the beginning of the nineteenth century, work was recognised for its curative effect and patients took an active part in the various industrial activities of each hospital, such as the kitchens, laundry, wards, dining halls, farm, garden, grounds, etc., still the work attaching to these various departments was not planned on a definite therapeutic basis and could only be described as 'industrial occupations.' The primary therapeutic purpose became submerged by the more attractive economic aspect and the affected patients were only considered in terms of the reduction of hospital costs. Even thus, while in individual cases, some therapeutical benefits may have accrued, there was no system of application, no consideration for the individual interests of the patients concerned, in relation to the work undertaken. There was no organisation, or scheme, prescribed, applied and supervised. There was, in fact, no occupational therapy properly so called, as we now know it. This was, unfortunately, the position right through the nineteenth century in all mental hospitals and was referred to specially by Dr. Frank Hoyt, Superintendent of the Iowa State Mental Hospital in a paper read at a meeting of the American Medico-Psychological Association in 1898. The following is an extract from Dr. Hoyt's remarks:

'Notwithstanding that, for half a century, the superintendents of our American Hospitals for the insane have had their attention called repeatedly to the "occupation treatment of the insane," the fact remains that . . . far too many can report no greater diversity of employment, nor more methodical application of this form of treatment, than was done fifty years ago. That this state of affairs exists is not due to any serious doubts as to the value of this method of treatment, but, rather, to an imperfect appreciation of its inestimable value, regardless of its economic features. The rock on which is wrecked many a newly launched ship of industrial treatment is that of Economy. Does it pay is the question most frequently asked by visitors to our industrial department. As well might one ask does it pay to use the knife, administer drugs, provide skilled nurses and the various paraphernalia of a well-organised hospital. Industrial treatment of the insane does pay . . . properly administered, it pays enormous profits in evidence in the wards of the hospital.'

To Dr. Simon of Germany must be given primary credit for the utilisation of occupations, both the industrial occupations prevailing in every mental hospital and special handicrafts, on a definite system and plan, based on curative end-results only. It was in 1905 in the Westphalian State Mental Hospital at Gutersloh, situated between Dusseldorf and Hanover, that Simon evolved his scheme of occupational therapy and applied it systematically throughout the entire hospital. The energy and success of his efforts may be gauged from the fact that he succeeded in occupying, in a therapeutic sense, 98% of his patients. His reputation spread, not only to other mental hospitals in Germany, but throughout Europe generally. Simon's methods were successfully copied at the State Hospital of Baden, at Richenau and also at the South German Mental Hospital at Constanz, as well as many others.

Although, as stated already, occupations were availed of in nearly all mental hospitals on an industrial basis, almost since their inception, it was not till subsequent to the 1914-18

War that they began to be organised under the term 'occupational therapy.' This title appears to have been first used by a Chicago man of Irish extraction, named George Edward Barton, when giving a name to his method of treating arthritic conditions by special occupational exercises, sometime about the year 1912.

Following on the success of the various 'ward aides' from England, Canada and America, in dealing with the sick and disabled soldiers during and after the 1914-18 War, occupational therapy received its first correct directional inspiration in America and Canada. During the War, special war-service courses, of the short, intensive type, were arranged at different centres to meet the demands for 'aides,' who were subsequently styled 'occupational therapists.' A number of such training courses had been in operation at a few centres in America prior to the War, and probably the first of its kind was that organised as a Summer course in 1909 by the Chicago School of Civics and Philanthropy. Owing to the War impetus and the establishment of these lightning courses, there was a rapid graduation of occupational therapists in America. This led to the establishment of a central organisation, when the American Occupational Therapy Association was created in 1917, one of the founders of which was its late Secretary-Treasurer, Mrs. Eleanor Clarke-Slagle, who was the originator of the special habit-training programme for mental cases, which is referred to later, in detail. Due to the energetic, collective activities of this body, training programmes were standardised and occupational therapy was placed on a properly-planned systematic basis to meet the needs and requirements of the various hospitals and institutions, covering Mental, General, Orthopaedic, Tubercular, Children's Hospitals, as well as Correctional Institutions and Mental Defective Colonies, involving the employment of over 1,000 occupational therapists. Some hospitals provided out-patient workshops, notably at the Vanderbilt Clinic of the Medical Centre, New York. In the Montefiore Hospital, where chronic conditions, covering tubercular, neurological, medical and surgical cases, are dealt with, occupational treatment was

applied under the supervision of several occupational
therapists.

In February, 1922, the American Occupational Therapy
Association sponsored the publication of a bi-monthly
magazine devoted solely to occupational treatment and
rehabilitation. One of its founders and first editor was
Dr. William R. Dunton, jr., who steered it from success
to success for an uninterrupted period of over 20 years.
After twenty-five years, this magazine was taken over by
the publishers and edited by the Association as *The American
Journal of Occupational Therapy*. These journals, together
with small magazines issued by local groups and the general
work of the Association, have done much to advance a
knowledge of, and the benefits to be attained by, the use
of occupational therapy.

All these activities in the U.S.A. brought the treatment
to the forefront of therapeutics and helped to have it recognised as a science, in its own right.

In Canada, the story of rapid post-war development is
very much akin to that in the United States. During the
1914-18 War, Canada, too, was one of the first countries
to organise occupational therapy on a definitely curative
basis. The late Mr. T. B. Kidner of Ottawa, who has written
an extremely interesting booklet on occupational therapy,
was appointed by the United States, shortly after their
entry into the War, to organise occupational treatment in
their military hospitals. In 1918 in Canada, it was decided
to establish six weeks' courses to provide sufficient of these
'aides,' as they were then called, and the urgency of the
matter had, of necessity, to override questions of academic
qualifications, age, experience, etc. Only girls possessing
'charm' were allowed for training. Dealing with this matter
at the time, Professor Haultain, Vocational Officer for the
Ontario Department of Soldiers' Civil Re-establishment,
said: 'Charm does not mean feminine beauty. We were sure
that, if we liked them, the soldiers would like them.' Two
hundred of these aides were trained, even though hastily,
and, following on the success of their efforts during the
War, the necessity for banding themselves into a single

organisation became an accomplished fact in 1920, when
the Ontario Society of Occupational Therapy was established
under the guidance of Dr. Goldwin Howland, whose name
was subsequently associated with the presidency of the
Canadian Association of Occupational Therapy. The movement spread through the mental hospitals, military hospitals
and general hospitals. The Toronto General Hospital
established an occupational therapy department. The
standardisation of the training courses under medical direction
became a problem to ensure that occupational therapists
should have a high standard of education as a basis for
training. Through Dr. Howland's representations to the
Toronto University authorities, a two-years' course in the
University was established.

It is, therefore, to the laudable efforts of the Canadian
enthusiasts that, in 1925, the first university course of its
kind was established to further the study of occupational
treatment. It has given to occupational therapy an educational
standing, which is only in keeping with the dignified and
important position that such a humane movement should
occupy. As a professional body, the necessity for a national
organisation, with a national register, was responsible for
the establishment of the Canadian Association of Occupational
Therapy in 1926, which published a quarterly journal.
Since then, the success of the movement has been signalised
by the founding of occupational therapy departments in the
Royal Victoria Hospital, Montreal; the Toronto East General
Hospital and the Sick Children's Hospital, Toronto, while
the Vancouver General Hospital has now two workshops,
one for general cases and the other for tubercular cases.
Tribute must undoubtedly be paid to both Canada and the
United States of America for the forward development
of present-day occupational therapy. Standards of training
and efficiency of method have been set as a headline to be
emulated by other countries. The primary therapeutic
purpose has been kept to the forefront and sound principles
in both training and application have been and are being
inculcated at all occupational centres. While the position
in other countries must be governed and regulated by local

conditions and circumstances, one would like to see occupational therapy given due recognition through properly accepted university standards of training and the extension of the treatment to the therapeutic departments of all hospitals, covering both mental and physical maladies.

Passing from the American Continent to Europe, we find that, with the exception of Germany, where, as already mentioned, Dr. Simon introduced his pioneer methods, which were successfully operated throughout Germany, occupational treatment on therapeutic lines was a post-war (1914-18) development and, in many cases, of very recent origin. The success of the work in German mental hospitals spread to some of the hospitals for disabled children and cripples. The Cripples' Hospital at Volksdorf, Hamburg, had one of the most up-to-date therapeutic workshops of its kind, with special sections for the young. Remedial exercises were provided for in a specially equipped gymnasium and in special diving baths. The following list of crafts indicates the novel type of work undertaken: shoemaking and repairs, manufacture of celluloid goods and bandages, smith work, plating and nickelling, including metal polishing, etc. In the Humanitas Hospital for crippled children in Saxony, occupational therapy workshops were provided with central playrooms on each floor and a large, fully-equipped chemical laboratory, providing advanced instruction for suitable patients.

It was not till 1926 that Holland introduced occupational therapy into the mental hospitals, following on the training of 60 nurses from Santpoort Mental Hospital, Amsterdam, at Dr. Simon's hospital at Gutersloh. The work was developed as at Gutersloh, but it was found necessary to introduce, in addition to members of the existing nursing staff, technicians who had no nursing qualifications or experience, but who were capable of teaching more advanced handicrafts. Lectures, demonstrations and handicraft training were included in the curriculum of the probationers' course in addition to the ordinary nursing requirements. Occupations were taught in each ward and in central workshops, where advanced handicrafts were organised under the supervision of the technicians.

In Switzerland, the Simon method was introduced into the Burgholzli Mental Hospital at Zurich in 1930 and to a number of other institutions, where the curative value of occupations was recognised as a supplemental aid to the existing methods of treatment. In the various tubercular sanatoria, occupational therapy is a prominent feature. A rather unique and important application of the treatment was developed in the Leysin International Sun Hospital under the famous Dr. Rollier, originator of the method. This consists of a simultaneous use of occupational therapy and heliotherapy. The occupations are carried through during graduated exposure to the sun. Speaking of this, Dr. Rollier says:—

'We endeavour to develop the specific resistance of every patient, concomitantly with his general resistance, by encouraging the practice of manual work, progressively and carefully adapted to each individual. The work cure is, of course, carried on in the sun whenever possible.'

The work performed is mostly of the mechanical type, such as the manufacture of induction coils, clock parts, metal parts and the assembling and finishing of clocks. The work attaching to the completion of each article is graded to meet the output ability associated with each type of tubercular condition. Induction coils are wound and finished by a number of bedridden patients, each making his own special contribution to the assembly, simulating a mass-production arrangement. The workshops are utilised by the convalescent type of patient, as he graduates from the ward occupations. Due to the success of the work treatment at Leysin, the general hospitals throughout Switzerland were mainly influenced in inaugurating occupational therapy departments and the movement spread generally through the country.

In Great Britain, occupational therapy has, for long, been availed of in the treatment of tuberculosis and mental deficiency. Among the former may be mentioned the Papworth Colony, Malting's Farm Sanatorium, Nayland, and Preston Hall, Maidstone. In these, as in all other sanatoria, the occupational work is under medical direction and applied to meet the individual needs of the patient and his condition. The treatment, generally, is based on rest and graduated exercise, the latter consisting of a combination of walking and working. A variety of occupations is utilised, the range differing in the many sanatoria. The Papworth Colony, which is self-supporting, was noted for the manufacture of leather cases and trunks, many of which were exported to foreign markets. In the mental deficiency colonies, occupational treatment is highly developed, interspersed, as it should be, with a vocational and economic element, so desirable in the socialisation of the many different types of ailments requiring treatment. A visit to the Manor Park, Epsom, or the Darenth Colony in Kent will demonstrate the extent and type of occupations in use. In these will be seen brushcraft, woodworking, bookbinding and printing, stitchcraft, weaving, rugmaking, etc. A novel feature in another of these colonies is the establishment of a special farm unit, where a number of high grade defectives live and dine in a self-contained farmhouse at some distance from the main institution. They are given special concessions and payment, which appear to instil a good deal of self-confidence and a most socialising sense of ownership.

Notwithstanding the pioneer work of Tuke at the Retreat, York, who stressed the therapeutic advantages of work for mental cases, occupational treatment in Great Britain generally did not come fully under the influence of the German example of Dr. Simon until following a visit to the Dutch Mental Hospitals and Clinics, organised by the Royal-Medico-Psychological Association in 1928.

The following hospitals were visited: Santpoort, Maasoord, Apeldoorn, Brinkgreven, Den Dolder and Bloemendaal, as well as a number of mental clinics. Dr. A. E. Evans, in his report of the Tour, stated:—

'Reviewing the journey, one must first record the deep impression of the thoroughness with which our Dutch colleagues apply the therapeutic and other principles of the soundness of which they are satisfied. The atmosphere of quiet industry, with the absence from the wards of noisy brawling or introspective idleness, in most of the hospitals we visited, has been a noteworthy achievement of painstaking labour.'

The patent success of occupational therapy in the Dutch

mental hospitals made an indelible impression on the members of the Tour, many of whom immediately faced the difficult task of introducing the treatment in their respective hospitals, notably at the Devon County Mental Hospital at Exminster, near Exeter, the North Riding Hospital at Clifton, Yorkshire, Cardiff City Mental Hospital, Severalls, Chester, Barming Heath and several others. The success of the movement in these latter hospitals constituted them as training centres, where many of the other mental hospitals sent some of their nurses to secure the necessary instruction for the establishment of treatment facilities in their own. Thus, in the post-war (1914-'18) years, great progress was made in Great Britain. A special training centre was established in the Dorset House School of Occupational Therapy at Clifton Down, Bristol. A two-years' course for resident women was given, consisting of lectures, demonstrations and practical training at Dorset House, as well as at the Bristol and Chester Mental Hospitals and other hospitals in the district. A similar non-resident course was available for men. Facilities for training were also made available at the London College for Nursing, in collaboration with the Maudsley Hospital and at Northampton, the Retreat, York, and at Liverpool and other centres. These centres were responsible for the graduation of a number of fully trained occupational therapists, which led to the establishment of The Association of Occupational Therapists in 1936.

This gradual development of training facilities, and the extension of the treatment in the various mental hospitals, aroused widespread interest, and quite a number of general and other hospitals have now introduced occupational therapy centres.

It is noteworthy that the first general impulse for the development of occupational therapy in Great Britain followed after the 1914-'18 war, when special treatment facilities had to be provided for wounded and disabled soldiers and sailors. This post-war stimulus was further reinforced by equally similar conditions succeeding the recent world war and rehabilitation centres were of general establishment. Referring to these latter in the *British Medical Journal* in

1943, Dr. G. R. Girdlestone, the then President of the British Orthopaedic Association, is quoted, as follows:—

'I think we all feel that rehabilitation should begin very soon after the accident or wound and be carried on throughout the patient's period in Hospital in the form of Occupational Therapy and gymnastic or remedial exercises.'

This recommendation, even if confined to orthopaedics, is an indication of the gradual penetration of occupational therapy activities into all branches of medical therapeutics and is a strong pointer for future development and extension generally in Great Britain.

In Scotland, the position is somewhat similar to that in England and Wales. Occupational therapy is a feature of most mental hospitals, tubercular sanatoria, mental deficiency colonies and orthopaedic hospitals. A very forward and progressive step was taken at the Astley-Ainslie Institution, Edinburgh in 1933, when the services of an occupational therapist were secured to ensure the most modern and up-to-date form of the treatment. Miss Amy De Brisay, Chief of the Occupational Therapy Department of the Toronto General Hospital, Canada, was chosen for this pioneer missionary work. A central workshop was established with ramifications of the treatment in the different wards. Sound therapeutic principles were inculcated. The financial expenditure and returns were in no way allowed to interfere with the primary therapeutic purpose. The treatment was linked with the existing physiotherapy department, with each maintaining an autonomous independence under the medical superintendent's direction.

With the remarkable progress of the treatment in Great Britain generally, its universal adoption in the general hospitals on intensive lines has yet to await the conviction of the medical and other authorities. In the absence of a practical experience, there may be a tendency to regard it as a 'hospital frill' and an unjustifiable expenditure, but the doctor's troubles associated with the difficult period of convalescence in all hospitals can be resolved in the occupational therapy department as in no other way. This, with the assurance that the treatment tends to reduce the number of hospital days per patient, as well as many other proven advantages, should justify a fair trial for the treatment in all the general hospitals.

In Italy, occupational therapy is of more recent origin in the mental hospitals and was not introduced into the chief mental hospital in Rome until 1931. Its recognition as a treatment was also a post-war (1914-'18) innovation, when the question of the rehabilitation of the wounded and disabled soldiers became an acute problem. This was largely solved by the establishment of workshops or, as they were called 'Clinics of Work.' The largest workshop of this kind was situated in Milan, which showed the influence of American teaching.

In Denmark, occupational treatment is a feature of most of the mental hospitals and is based on the usual accepted practice, including the mental deficiency institutions. Remedial occupations are also operated in the tubercular sanatoria and are developed on vocational, as well as therapeutic lines.

In France, occupational treatment is practised in a large number of the mental hospitals, as well as in the tubercular sanatoria and hospitals for crippled children. Apart from the use of remedial occupations at Vittel and Vichy, the treatment has not, otherwise, extended to the general and convalescent hospitals and does not appear to have found favour, generally, with the physicians and surgeons of these hospitals.

In Ireland, the position outlined in Great Britain is somewhat similar. Occupational treatment has, for a long number of years, been a feature of some of the tubercular sanatoria, the orphanages, blind asylums and the mental deficiency institutions. At the Peamount Sanatorium, Dublin, occupational therapy led to the development of the famous Peamount Industries, which, mostly confined to woodworking, have proved a very successful follow-up treatment in the convalescent period of tuberculosis. The occupations available are utilised for both therapeutic and vocational reasons. Some of the patients have been retained in permanent employment after recovery.

In the mental hospitals, though special occupations, such

as weaving, basketry, brushcraft, mat-making, upholstery, etc., have been in use for a number of years, even prior to the 1914-'18 War, these have been based more on the economic requirements of the hospitals. They have been supervised by paid tradesmen, with a limited number of assisting patients, whose therapeutic requirements were not given due consideration. These, as in Canada and the United States before the Great War and in Great Britain prior to 1929, were mainly industrial occupations subserving economic interests. In 1934, occupational therapy departments were established in the Killarney Mental Hospital, and in a number of the other mental hospitals throughout the country.

The treatment in Killarney Mental Hospital is based on a combination of the Simon system and American-Canadian practice. The services of occupational therapists have not been sought, the work being undertaken by the more skilled members of the nursing staffs, special efforts being made to extend the treatment to the more restless and excited patients. In addition to ward occupations, special occupational centres have been established for more advanced work. In Killarney Mental Hospital, the daily percentage occupied of the total number of patients, including those acutely ill, ranges from 85% to 90%. The development of many special craft centres throughout both the male and female sides of the hospital, as well as re-education therapy classes and recreational treatment centres, has facilitated follow-up treatment in all cases submitted for insulin therapy and electro-convulsant treatment. All patients, as soon as they exhibit a positive response to the latter physical methods of treatment, are immediately submitted, under prescription card, for appropriate occupational treatment. This has an additional reinforcing value in the physical treatments, which tends to speed up, in a very appreciable manner, the period of recovery in all the favourable cases.

It is hoped that the recognition of this reinforcement factor in occupational therapy will help to convince the responsible administrators of all hospitals, including the general hospitals, of the advantages of establishing occupational therapy centres as a standard form of treatment. The university authorities might, likewise, be influenced in providing suitable courses of training, so as to produce fully certificated occupational therapists. These therapists would, thus, be qualified to promote, on a scientific and high level, the establishment of complete occupational therapy facilities in every type of hospital throughout the country.

# CHAPTER III.

## PRINCIPLES, RULES, OBJECTS AND ADVANTAGES

### PRINCIPLES AND RULES OF OCCUPATIONAL THERAPY

OCCUPATIONAL THERAPY, as a science, must have definite basic principles and rules of guidance for its practical application in its various branches. Whether in psychological or general medicine or in surgery, or in any of the special branches, it may become necessary to develop for each, special rules of guidance, but all must be governed by the general principles underlying any successful application of the treatment. These general principles are formulated on a *sine qua non* basis and must be given full cognisance for a proper and successful issue in all cases. Failure to keep these principles in view must, of necessity, result in failure to achieve the end-results aimed at. The principles are essential, the rules of guidance are merely additional desiderata, which an industrious and painstaking nurse or occupational therapist will recognise and apply to secure the best results.

1. *Occupational Therapy is primarily a form of treatment.*

This is the basic and one of the most important principles of occupational therapy. An analysis of the principle shows that O.T. is a definite therapeusis or treatment and is described as occupational, as it utilises various occupations and handicrafts, purely and primarily for their curative effect. Being essentially a treatment or curative agent, it should be regarded in the light of all other forms of therapy, as a definite expenditure securing very definite practical results. It should be completely measured by its therapeutic results and its cost and financial considerations should be subordinated thereto. It is exceedingly difficult to secure the wholehearted co-operation of the lay-mind in this direction when establishing an occupational therapy department in any type of hospital. The inclination to give chief thought to the expenditure and possible financial returns, to the exclusion of what should be the primary consideration, namely, the curative results to be attained, is an obstacle which generally has to be surmounted.

The various forms of physiotherapy, hydrotherapy, electrotherapy, etc., have now found a place in the therapeutic equipment of all modern hospitals. Their installation and annual working costs, as in all other forms of hospital therapy, have been justified on their curative results. Their utilisation by the hospital staff is, in no way, governed from the financial standpoint. Occupational therapy, which is closely allied to physiotherapy and, in some hospitals, housed in the same section, is, unfortunately, not always given the same considerations. Its economic possibilities as a useful adjunct in meeting hospital expenditure is often its chief recommendation to its establishment in the first instance. Subsequently, this consideration tends to relegate to the background its primary purpose, even sometimes in medical minds. Unless the therapeutic aspect is kept to the forefront and is, in fact, the sole guiding factor, then this form of treatment changes from occupational therapy to industrial occupation—a position which should not prevail in any hospital where the principles of occupational therapy are fully recognised.

The vital importance of this basic principle may be gauged by analogical comparison. The curative aspect is to occupational therapy what the soul is to the body. It is the vital principle, which gives life and without which the treatment is no longer a treatment—it is merely an inanimate body, which is devitalised, inert and useless. The soul or therapy is gone and the lifeless body or occupation is all that remains. Therefore, in any branch of occupational therapy, properly so-called, the curative aspect must, at all times, be kept to the forefront. It must be the chief consideration and all others must be secondary and in no way interfere with this primary purpose.

The recognition of this principle, however, does not create a prescriptive right to exclude all other considerations in the operation of the treatment. As in other forms of therapy and hospital administration, due regard and attention must be paid to the economic side. Unnecessary waste must be avoided and the standard of production must aim at optimum results. The sales and purchases sections of the department must be organised on up-to-date business lines, the importance of which will be dealt with fully in a later chapter. By paying due regard to this aspect of the question and without minimising the proper import or in any way losing sight of the primary and basic principle of occupational therapy, enunciated above, it is possible to make the department, at the least, self-supporting.

2. *The Treatment must, at all times, be under expert medical direction.*

This principle postulates an important condition for its scientific application. Just as the various therapeutic departments of every hospital are under medical control, so, likewise, with occupational therapy. In addition, just as each of the former is supervised by a medical expert in his respective branch, the occupational therapy department must also have expert medical direction. The medical superintendent, in taking supreme control, must have made a special study of the subject. He must be versed in the various details of organisation, with its ramifications in the wards, special occupational centres, workshops, etc. He must, in fact, be acquainted in, at least, a general way, with both the theory and practice of the treatment. This will be necessary for the proper allocation of duties to his various medical officers. The latter, in turn, will be required to take charge of various sections and must, likewise, possess the necessary qualifications to ensure the success of the treatment and its harmonious progress in the different sections. They must be in the position to prescribe the correct type of occupation in each individual case and note the progress of each case. They must prescribe and supervise the social and recreational side—a very important branch of the treatment. They have, in fact, many functions to perform, to be dealt with in a later chapter, which indicate the necessity for a thorough experience and practical knowledge of O.T. in all its forms.

3. *Occupational Therapy must be evolved on a definite system and applied methodically.*

The diversity of the available occupations and handicrafts, as well as the variability of the patients recommended for treatment, whether on mental or physical grounds, necessitate that occupational therapy should be built on a definite system and avail of precise and ordered methods of procedure. This must, obviously, be a basic principle of any form of treatment and is essential in occupational therapy as in all other forms of therapeusis. Unless our methods of treatment are definite and precise, we cannot hope to secure the results anticipated. Ward occupations must be organised systematically to take cognisance of the necessity for bedside occupations, dayroom occupations and the provision of a ward occupational room, where possible. The type of patients undergoing treatment will vary according to the ward. The reception wards will require special consideration, as distinct from the chronic or other wards. The organisation of special occupational centres and the linking up of the existing workshops will all be based on a definite system. Likewise, the personnel of the system, from the superintendent right down to the junior nurse associated with the treatment, must also be arranged in a definite manner, where each member will be duly aware of his individual *locus standi* and the contribution which each must make to ensure the correct *modus operandi* of the treatment, as well as the attainment of the desired end-results. All these points will be dealt with in detail later, according as they arise. It is sufficient here to refer to them in a general way to indicate the necessity for recognising this very important principle.

4. *The Patient's Competence and Interests must be considered in relation to the work to be prescribed.*

This principle, while chiefly of medical interest, also comes within the purview of the occupational therapist,

who is the officer in charge of the entire occupational department, and, as it were, the liaison officer between the medical
staff and the actual working details of the treatment. The
first important point emanating from this principle is that no
occupation should be prescribed that is obviously beyond
the patient's capacity for performance, or of a type incapable
of stimulating or maintaining his interest. This might,
possibly, arise on mental grounds as well as physical. The
advanced dement, whose range of work does not extend
beyond rag-teasing and similar simple tasks, would be
completely outside the ambit of occupational therapy if
directed to take charge of a pedal loom. Conversely, the
medical officer prescribing for the convalescent manic-
depressive, the sanding of wooden toys, the assembly of
which are more within his competence and obvious interests,
displays a definite lack of appreciation of the principles and
practice of the treatment.

In addition to grading the occupation to the patient's
ability and competence, consideration must also be given
to his expressed or estimated interests. If the work prescribed
does not prove congenial and make a personal appeal to
the patient, then it resolves itself into an undesirable task
that has to be performed, somehow. Fatigue and ennui
will replace the delight and satisfaction that should normally
ensue in performing and completing the work. The therapeutic effect aimed at will be nullified and the possibility
of negativism and other objectionable traits, making their
appearance, may add to the difficulties of the situation.
In addition, the usual beneficial environmental influence
of a special occupational therapy section may be permanently
counteracted and such an adverse first impression may do
incalculable harm, lasting weeks or even months. A reverse
of this kind dealt out to a patient in the early stages of his
illness, even unintentionally, may defeat all the benefits
and objects of occupational treatment.

The recognition of this principle involves, not alone a
grading or classification of the patients to be treated, but,
also, a grading of the various occupations and handicrafts.
The latter have to be studied and understood from the point

of view of their interest motivation in relation to the various psychological types to be treated. A proper medical diagnosis in each case must be co-ordinated with the intellectual, emotional and volitional tendencies, to ascertain the work capacity and the range of interests, with a view to prescribing the correct occupation. An incorrect diagnosis, in the first instance, will inevitably lead to a faulty prescription and ultimately to negative results. Neglect to estimate the intellectual capacity will result in recommending an unsuitable occupation. A person of low or even moderate intellectual attainments cannot be expected to perform work that is obviously beyond his powers of comprehension. For the same reason, such work cannot lie within the range of his estimated interests and would, in this way, be an additional violation of the principle. Due regard must also be paid to the patient's emotional content. The hilarious, euphoric patient requires a more sedative type of occupation to allay excitement than the depressed type, whose movements are confined to the terminal joints. Both cases will require persistent supervision, the former for mutability of attention and the latter for retardation; the interest displayed in both cases being governed by the strength and concentration of attention present.

The volitional attitude of the patient must also be discerned from the outset to secure his proper co-operation. Compulsion or coercion of any kind must never be resorted to. Through persuasion and inducement lie the only permissible methods of approach to convince the patient of the therapeutic necessity of the treatment. Frank discussion must take place to assure him that, while the work to be performed may be of economic value to the hospital, its primary motive is to benefit his own individual health and promote the collective comfort and well-being of the hospital community. Katatonic negativism, melancholic resistiveness and hebephrenic aloofness will be some of the volitional traits among many other obstacles that will have to be surmounted in the initial stages. If these are not recognised, through imperfect examination or faulty diagnosis, the resulting incorrect prescription will only add to the difficulties of the occupational therapist. The latter's task in dealing with each type of case just quoted, even when correctly diagnosed, is, at all times, a most arduous one, often resulting in initial failure.

The approach to the patient should be such as to arouse not only his interest but his confidence. This may have to extend beyond the first initial discussion and several interviews may be necessary to effect this. He should be accepted in the role of an essential and much appreciated assistant to the staff in charge of the work. An atmosphere of equality should prevail in all departments, where the patient should be made to feel that his contribution ranks of equal importance with the supervisory duties of the attending nurse or the occupational therapist. The factory atmosphere, where the directors have only a limited contact with the workers, must never make its appearance in an occupational therapy department. This sense of equality has a most beneficial environmental influence, tending to promote confidence and maintain the patient's interest.

It will be seen, therefore, that the principle we are discussing, dealing as it does with the patient's competence and interests, has a very wide application. It includes the regulation and grading of the work prescribed to allow for the growing interests and the increasing strength and ability of the patient. In this way, the monotony of a continued succession of simple movements, the accomplishment of which, in the early stages, may meet the needs of the case, is obviated by a scheme of grading and promotion to more complicated and absorbing work.

5. *Occupational Therapy should exhibit diversity and novelty in all its forms of activity.*

The operation of this principle is essential for the harmonious and successful working of the treatment and is applicable, not alone to the handicrafts availed of, but, also, to the recreational and social forms of the therapy. It presupposes a well-balanced programme of work, rest and exercise to be arranged daily. This is easily catered for in the mental hospitals, where the variety and novelty associated with the routine functions of hospital life are further enhanced by the addition of special crafts. The former range from the work on the farm, garden and grounds to the laundry, wards, kitchen and other utility services, in addition to the different trades shops. The latter, including the standard crafts of weaving, woodcraft and basketry, may be supplemented by a host of major and minor occupations. All these, on the occupational side, furnish the novelty and variety that are a feature of occupational therapy departments in mental hospitals and are further enhanced by the addition of social and recreational activities.

On the other hand, in orthopaedic, general and most convalescent hospitals, the facilities outlined are not available to the same extent and the occupational departments in these hospitals are more limited in the number of crafts utilised, as well as the recreational and social activities available. It is in these hospitals that the recognition of the principle calls for most attention, where the ingenuity and resourcefulness of the occupational therapist will be taxed in its observance. The range and variety of the crafts will be increased to the maximum permitted by space and other considerations. The recreational and social side will provide for as much novelty and diversity as may be permissible. This will increase the treatment facilities of the department and cover the wide occupational needs of all its patients.

6. *The Treatment is only to be judged by its effect on the patient in each case, whether the products show inferior workmanship or not.*

This principle indicates that the patient and the effects of the treatment take priority over the quality of the articles produced, as well as their output and saleability. If the work prescribed is not having the desired results, then the prescription requires amending. The work itself may be at fault, or the environment, or method of the work. Some patients respond to the treatment more rapidly in group occupations rather than when working alone. Others fail to maintain the necessary interest unless executing work unaided. They lose the sense of accomplishment, so essential in securing the beneficial effects of the treatment, when participating in group or collective occupations. Thus, the individual needs in each case must be studied and considered in planning suitable occupation. The type of work recommended, too, is of vast importance. In some cases the best results are attained by outdoor occupations and the large variety of the latter require consideration in each case. Others give the best results when working indoors, due allowance being paid in planning the health needs of such cases.

The standard of the work performed must not be set as a criterion of the results aimed at. What might be regarded as simple or trivial to the normal, may produce beneficial results in the case of those mentally or physically ill. The winding of a ball of wool may meet the occupational needs of a case in the early stages of his disease, when the same case, with improving health and interests, may peg the same type of wool on the warping frame without missing a count. Similarly, the finishing of a misshapen and ungainly-looking wicker basket may have more therapeutic possibilities for the patient concerned than the creation of a beautifully finished coloured flower basket in another case. Nevertheless, the aim at all times must be toward the best finish for each article, as the stimulation to normal standards begets confidence and arouses hope. The creation of normal standards in work suggests the approach to normal health in people, who may have lost faith in themselves. They cannot be but beneficially influenced at the realisation of their restored ability to accomplish something useful and worth while. The mental satisfaction and stimulation that is normally associated with the accomplishment of any useful task can only be measured in a relative manner in the case of the mentally abnormal or even the physically disabled, when completing such a task. Based even on such relative standards of measurement, it can be readily seen what a tremendous therapeutic force, properly directed occupation can be, for the mentally and physically ill.

7. *The Occupational Therapist must have the necessary technical knowledge, special aptitude for imparting instruction, and a suitable temperament and manner.*

The occupational therapist, as already pointed out, is the senior officer immediately responsible to the medical officer in charge and the medical superintendent for the working and success of the entire occupational therapy department. To ensure the proper and successful functioning of the department, he must have the necessary qualifications, technical and otherwise. He must, in other words, have undergone a special course of training, at a recognised centre, and qualified as such. He must have attained a sound knowledge of the details of all the handicrafts associated with the treatment. In addition, he must have studied the necessary psychology and benefited from such study. He must have acquired a general knowledge of mental diseases, including the various clinical and psychological states suitable for occupational treatment. He must, in fact, be an expert in the theory and practice of occupational therapy.

It is not sufficient to be versed in the theory and practice of the treatment, the capacity to teach and instruct is also an important essential. The elementary as well as the intricate details of the different crafts will have to be demonstrated and explained, not alone to the patients submitted for treatment, but also to the nursing staff, who are to assist in the work. Failure to make these details explicit and intelligible, due to absence of the necessary special ability on the part of the therapist, will militate against the success of the department. This will result in a tendency to confuse rather than enthuse the patient, with consequent depreciation of interest and lack of confidence, so detrimental to his receptive faculties. The therapeutic and other progress of the case will be materially affected and the results anticipated will not be realised.

In addition to the academic qualifications, which, as outlined, are vitally essential, there are personality qualifications of equal importance. Just as the nurse requires certain general qualifications to be fitted for the post of nursing, so, also, the occupational therapist must possess a suitable disposition and manner to attain the correct contact with his patients. The correct temperament is as necessary for success as the profundity of knowledge. A cheerful and prepossessing manner goes a long way to secure the patient's confidence and arouse his courage and ambition. The therapist who radiates cheerfulness in his department is destined to have the best and most rapid results. He must display tact and unbounded energy in his work, avoiding displays of ill-temper and any appearances of indolence or indifference. Proper planning and outlining of the day's work must be made in advance to avoid flurry and the possibility of 'crankiness' when anything goes wrong. But above all, forbearance and perseverance would appear to be the most essential possessions in the personality treasury of the therapist. These presuppose a sense of understanding and appreciation of the patient's ability and powers of reception. They provide, in full, for the failures that are inevitably encountered and make up for the deficiencies in progress that are the rule in many cases and help to tide the therapist over the most arduous and difficult portions of his task. The will to persevere against such difficulties must be ever present, as the patience required to overcome many trying situations will be taxed to the utmost. Otherwise, despair and indifference will be substituted and feelings such as these should never be exhibited in any occupational therapy department.

Many lines could be expended in appraising the character requirements of the occupational therapist, which might appear to aim at an almost impossible ideal. Still, certain standards must be laid down to which each therapist must aspire in order to approach this ideal. It is in striving for it that success is generally attained and there is no therapist, worthy of the name, who will not endeavour to reach the highest standards, which should characterise the profession.

These are the seven basic principles of occupational therapy which constitute the essential requirements for the treatment.

They will be supplemented in further chapters by subsidiary principles and rules of guidance in the various branches as they arise. These basic principles are essential in all forms and sections of the therapy. They apply to the handicraft, social and recreational activities of the treatment, whether availed of in mental disease, tuberculosis, amentia, orthopaedics, in general or convalescent hospitals. Each of the latter may require to formulate, in its respective branch, subsidiary principles and rules, but all are governed by the seven main principles.

The American Occupational Therapy Association has drafted a number of principles and rules for guidance, most of which are incorporated in the seven general principles already described. These run, as follows:—

1. Occupational therapy is a method of treatment of the sick or injured by means of purposeful occupation.

2. The objects sought are to arouse interest, courage and confidence; to exercise mind and body in healthy activity; to overcome disability and to re-establish capacity for industrial and social usefulness.

3. In applying occupational therapy, system and precision are as important as in other forms of treatment.

4. The treatment should be prescribed and administered under constant medical advice and supervision and correlated with the other treatment of the patient.

5. The treatment should, in each case, be specifically directed to the individual needs.

6. Though some patients do best alone, employment in groups is usually advisable, because it provides exercise in social adaptation and the stimulating influence of example and comment.

7. The occupation selected should be within the patient's estimated interests and capability.

8. As the patient's strength and capability increase, the type and extent of occupation should be regulated and graded accordingly.

9. The only reliable measure of the treatment is the effect on the patient.

10. Inferior workmanship, or employment in an occupation which would be trivial for the healthy, may be attended with the greatest benefit to the sick or injured, but standards worthy of entirely normal persons must be maintained for proper mental stimulation.

11. The production of a well-made, useful and attractive article, or the accomplishment of a useful task, requires healthy exercise of mind and body, gives the greatest satisfaction and thus produces the most beneficial effects.

12. Novelty, variety, individuality and utility of the products enhance the value of an occupation as a treatment measure.

13. Quality, quantity and saleability of the products may prove beneficial by satisfying and stimulating the patient, but should never be permitted to obscure the main purpose.

14. Good craftsmanship and ability to instruct are essential qualifications in the occupational therapist; understanding, sincere interest in the patient, and an optimistic, cheerful outlook and manner are equally essential.

15. Physical exercises, games and music are useful forms of occupational therapy and fall under two heads:—

A. Gymnastics and calisthenics that are given for their value in a patients' physical re-education, or in habit-training in mental hospitals.

B. Recreation and play activities, such as music, games, folk-dancing, etc., which are provided because of their general and social value for the patients.

At the 1930 International Congress on Mental Hygiene in Washington, U.S.A., Dr. Simon, of Gutersloh, Germany, read a short paper on his occupational method, from which the following is an abstract of the principles formulated by him:—

'1. Every achievement expected from the patient must remain within his capability, which must be determined exactly by the physician and nurse, because demands that are beyond his limitations cause, not only disagreeableness, dissatisfaction and opposition, but also inner unrest, fear and feelings of inferiority. All components of the total personality must here be considered; strength, versatility, responsiveness, co-ordination of thought, alertness and memory; likewise, also, the degree of impairment which all these capabilities have suffered from the disease.

2. The work must always be kept at the highest level of the patient's work efficiency, because the available energy can be strengthened only by its full utilization.

3. The constancy of the work assigned, facilitates the adjustment through practice and habituation which are powerful allies of therapy.

4. The work must be serious—no pastime or joke.

5. As many diverse forms of activity as possible should be available in all institutions.

6. No indolent loafing, with its evil consequences, should be tolerated.

7. Academic instruction, gymnastics, sports, rhythmic exercises and singing classes can also support the therapy.

8. Stimulation must come from the environment, the physician, the nurse, the other patients. Only by becoming once more accustomed to the fulfilment of duties can the patient rise to the level of an independent personality, thus preparing for his return into free communal and economic life.'

## Objects and Advantages of Occupational Therapy

The main object and purpose of occupational therapy is to secure recovery in the treatment of both mental and physical ailments. It should always be applied with this end in view, no matter how unfavourable the prognosis, in any individual case. The primary purpose of healing should be kept to the forefront even when it is obvious that the end-result in a particular case cannot possibly lead to complete recovery. Many psychotic and paralytic cases will be submitted for treatment, where complete recovery is out of the question, but, if any results are to be obtained in such cases, they must secure their motivating force through the influence and appeal to be derived from the guiding spirit of the main object.

The driving principle of the treatment should direct towards total recovery or, when unsuccessful, towards the secondary purpose of securing amelioration of the condition and thence to partial recovery. There are many psychological and orthopaedic conditions, where, owing to pathological and other processes, it is not possible to secure absolutely normal functioning. The most that can be expected is a partial improvement, no matter how large or small, and the attainment of such positive results is preferable to purely negative ones. It may mean, in many cases, all the difference between social dependence and independence in self-support, subsequently. There are many cases on record, especially in orthopaedic conditions, where occupational therapy has been the sole factor in rehabilitation to the extent of preventing such cases from being permanent state or family burdens. This is demonstrated in a remarkable way in the occupational and vocational treatment of congenital mental defectives (amentia).

A further object in occupational treatment, where both total and partial recovery are definitely impossible, occurs in arresting and preventing the regression associated with mental disease in its chronic stages. Many cases of schizophrenia lapse into varying stages of apparent mental deterioration if left untreated and not permitted to receive the advantages of remedial occupation; quite a large number, in fact, reach the profound type of regression associated with the 'wet and dirty' stage. The relative absence of this latter type of case in mental hospitals, where occupational therapy is practised in all its forms, bears definite evidence, if proof were needed, of the efficacy and influence of the treatment.

Even those cases, who have reached the 'wet and dirty' stage and whose habits are a constant source of worry to the medical and nursing staffs, may be retrieved and returned to normal and better habits, under the influence of a special section of the treatment, known as Re-educational Therapy. By means of a habit-training programme specially devised to secure the best results, this type of case is trained to co-operate and induce the restoration of normal behaviour in habits and conduct. Later, the habit of occupation is inculcated and, though of a minor and simple type in the early stages, it often progresses to more difficult and complicated tasks and, sometimes, it eventually paves the way to a definite remission of the mental state, that might not, otherwise, be regarded possible. In addition to the improvement and restoration of clean habits, the facilitation of control in excited and destructive cases is also secured. The problem of the restless and destructive cases is probably one of the chief bugbears of mental nursing and administration. The nightly destruction of clothing and furniture in mental hospitals, if not completely eliminated under the ameliorating influence of occupational therapy, is certainly diminished to an extraordinary degree. The dissipation of the useless energy displayed by restless and destructive cases is diverted into more utilitarian channels, by means of purposeful occupation and, generally, after a busy day, provides a more rational soporific than the nightly dose of sedative.

The advantages of occupational therapy may be discussed under three heads—(1) *Psychological*, (2) *Physical* and (3) *Economic*.

1. *Psychologically* or from the mental standpoint, the advantages are manifold and of paramount importance. From the earliest times, the psychological effect of work has been recognised. It is the chief activity of every normal person, who, at some time or another, has realised its advantages over periods of enforced idleness. Many people find comfort and solace in their work and daily avocation during periods of great stress or grief, while, on the other hand, the effect of unemployment in the post-war (1914-'18) world depression, roused many governments to take inordinate steps to combat the evil. The stabilising influence of work,

in ordinary daily life, must be a potent factor in treatment, when scientifically directed under expert supervision in states of abnormalcy. The psychological advantages are (a) *subjective* and (b) *objective*, the former covering the personal reactions and the latter detailing the benefits to the hospital and community in general.

(a) On the patient's side, occupational therapy provides a means of influencing the outlook on hospitalisation. The boredom associated with the hospital period of mental or physical disease is eradicated and replaced by new interests and hopes. Introspection and autistic activities, so undesirable in the progress of treatment, are substituted by occupational interests, which, even in group activities, create useful social contacts and help to restore the gregarious instinct so essential to community life.

The inspiration of hopefulness and self-confidence, so lacking in the invalid, receives a new and fresh impetus. The creative instinct, which has been man's greatest urge and which may become submerged in feelings of inferiority and self-imposed failure, is resuscitated and brought into play by the subtle influence of scientifically guided occupation. The feeling that something can be accomplished is revived and the worthwhile attitude towards life is restored to its former healthy position. New contacts of resocialisation are made which give fresh spur to dormant ambitions and strengthen the will to recover and resume communal activities. The sense of responsibility, which may have been vitiated by antisocial behaviour, receives a salutary tonic on the completion of an absorbing task. Many restored functions, in both mental and physical disease, following occupational treatment, in individual cases, will arouse additional emotional reactions, from which further appraisal may be accorded the treatment and grateful patients will pay added tribute to its beneficent advantages.

(b) *Objectively*, the most striking psychological benefit of occupational therapy is the altered atmosphere of the hospital, especially in the refractory wards. The noisy and turbulent movements are replaced by quiet industry and the whole tone of the institution undergoes a revolutionary change.

Mechanical restraint, seclusion and hypnotic drug treatment become practically non-existent and the patients present a more contented and cheerful appearance. The difficult task of nursing and behaviour control assumes less arduous proportions and the monotonous life of daily supervision is given a new zest and appeal, which can only be fully realised from a practical experience of this change. The increased industry and busy routine, in all sections of the hospital, create an infectious atmosphere of cheerfulness and happiness that reacts favourably towards recovery and a more enlightened nursing spirit, generally.

2. *Physically*, a properly planned programme of work, rest and exercise must, of necessity, improve the bodily health and create favourable interactions between mental and bodily processes, recognising the efficacy of the well-known hygienic apothem—*mens sana in corpore sano*—a healthy mind in a healthy body. The promotion of physical health must react favourably towards improved mentation. In the orthopaedic field, occupational treatment helps to build up wasted muscles and degenerated nerves, restoring function to muscles affected from disuse atrophy and re-habilitating injured joints and structures. It co-operates with physiotherapy in restoring normal movements in the case of fractured bones and helps to tide over the difficult and often prolonged period of convalescence in all such cases. It increases bodily resistance to disease and infection by toning up the blood circulation and other vital bodily systems.

3. *On the Economic side* its value to the hospital and, subsequently, to the community, while not being over-emphasised, must be a strong recommendation. In the recoverable cases, it definitely reduces the number of hospital days per patient, with a consequent reduction in the cost of treatment. For those who cannot be persuaded to judge the treatment from any but the financial aspect, this point should make an immediate appeal. Unfortunately, in the absence of a less materialistic attitude and a definite system of assessment of results, in possible therapeutic units, the lay-mind will always be so disposed.

Its economic benefit to the hospital is further advanced

by the reduction in the extent of the usual damage to clothing and furniture so prevalent in the refractory sections of mental hospitals. Laundry working and costs are similarly reduced by a noticeable decrease in the quantity of soiled bed and other clothing. The replacement of paid labour in the utility services of the hospital and in supplying its manifold needs must be an economic factor of vast budgetary importance. Further, the irrecoverable case, whose period of hospitalisation must be of a permanent nature, is converted from a dead liability to a definite or partial asset, though his position in the occupational department is not measured on such grounds. In mental deficiency colonies and in out-patient services, the vocational aspect of the treatment leads to communal saving on a hitherto unprecedented scale. All these points make economic claims, which are a definite recommendation for occupational treatment, but should only be subsidiary reasons for its establishment and continuation as a therapeutic régime.

Isolated experiences and special incidents may add to the number and confirm the claims, just made, on behalf of occupational treatment; still there are many critics who maintain that it is merely a hospital 'frill.' Some have been known to describe it as purely 'window-dressing,' but it is doubtful if this opinion was based on any extended practical experience of the treatment. There are others who, while approving of outdoor occupations and activities of all types, are totally opposed to indoor and special handicraft centres, except in the case of the disabled and crippled. This latter form of reasoning, pushed to its extremes, must decry any sort of indoor occupation, even for the sane and healthy. Just as the achievement of such an Utopia in this workaday world is not permitted by the exigencies and circumstances of life, so, likewise, occupational treatment must be based on practicable and practical considerations. No mental hospital, of any standing, could possibly absorb, in outdoor activities solely, more than 50% of those capable of being occupied, if restrictions of the kind suggested were imposed. Many indoor occupations are generally transferred to the open in favourable weather and, surely, it is more preferable to have the additional 50% of the patients suitably occupied, even indoor, than aimlessly moping around wards and dayrooms, as would be the case, because of winter and other weather restrictions, merely to satisfy fresh-air faddists.

On the other hand, eminent psychiatrists and authorities, both past and present, have paid unmistakable tribute to the advantages of the treatment and their pronouncements, some of which have already been quoted, nullify any criticisms that may be offered. In 1854, the famous Dr. Kirkbride, of the U.S.A., said:—

> 'Labour is one of our best remedies; it is as useful in improving the health of the insane as in maintaining that of the sane. It is one of the best anodynes for the nervous, it composes the restless and excited, promotes a good appetite and a comfortable digestion and gives sound and refreshing sleep to many who would, without it, pass wakeful nights.'

Many other striking recommendations of occupational treatment have been made in the past century, but none so forceful and so concise as that of the late Dr. Thomas W. Salmon of the U.S.A., who said:—

> 'Occupational Therapy will some day rank with anaesthetics in taking the suffering out of sickness and with antitoxins in shortening its duration. The greater part of the distress in chronic disease is mental and occupational therapy is, thus far, our only means of dealing with this factor.'

This laconic and sententious pronouncement might, with general approval, be accepted as the Charter of Occupational Therapy in the very wide domain of therapeutics.

# CHAPTER IV.

## CLASSIFICATIONS AND SUBDIVISIONS
### of
## OCCUPATIONAL THERAPY

IT WILL BE NOTED in the recommended definition of occupational therapy, that the treatment requires classification, and subdivision. Based on application, there are two main divisions of the therapy, depicting its use in (a) mental disease and (b) physical disease. Likewise, in type, the occupational side is described as physical or mental, social or recreational, placing no limitation to the quality of the occupation. The absorbing interest of a suitable book may have as high a therapeutic value as the tooling of the most intricately designed leather wallet. The occupation in the former is purely mental, requiring no unusual physical effort and eminently suitable where bodily exertion is contraindicated, just as a well-balanced 'talkie' programme contributes to the passive enjoyment of its audience, forming a special feature of many occupational therapy departments.

Occupation, on the physical side, is not confined to handicrafts and manual tasks; Habit-training and Re-education, together with active recreation and physical exercises of all kinds, contribute to the diversity of the treatment. There are, thus, three broad types of occupational treatment (1) *Handicraft*, (2) *Recreational* and (3) *Re-educational* or *Habit-Training*, all of which, combined with properly timed sleep and rest, make for the therapeutic balance so essential for treatment. (4) *A Commercial Section* of the treatment, concerning the business or economic aspect, is also differentiated and discussed in detail in Chapter 10.

1. *Handicraft*: This subdivision of occupational therapy has been described by many writers under the rather confusing title of 'Occupational.' Recreational therapy is also occupational, though distinct from the handicraft side in

its method and procedure. Both subdivisions are based on their occupational content and it is incorrect to classify exclusively the handicrafts or work proper as 'occupational therapy' for this reason.

The handicraft side of the treatment may be further subdivided into (a) *Special* and (b) *General*. The latter would include the work associated with the utility and maintenance services of the hospital and would be concerned, though to a limited extent, in some hospitals, with work connected with the farm, garden, upkeep of grounds, trades-men's shops, laundry, kitchen, dininghalls, wards, etc. The former consists of the special crafts and work over and above the maintenance services just mentioned. They may add to the utility services of the hospital by the manufacture and supply of articles required for use, such as brushes, baskets, mats, etc. They may, in fact, further avail of the tradeshops by supplementing the routine work of these departments. The carpenter's shop may be utilised for the development of a special wood-working section for the manufacture of wooden toys, stools, furniture, etc. Metal-work of a specialised type may be carried on in the engineering shop, availing of the smithy section when necessary, for the furtherance of the work.

The painting and enamelling of articles made in the woodworking section may be completed in the painter's shop. All this work being of a specialised nature should be distinguished from the general routine activities associated with the maintenance services of the hospital. It is impossible to give an exhaustive list of the crafts that may be organised in the special and other sections of an occupational therapy department, as local and individual circumstances may add to those generally in vogue. The following list, however, should cover the more usual types of crafts met with:—

*Stitchcraft*—Including sewing, knitting, lacework, tapestry, crochet, drawn-thread work, embroidery, quilting, etc.

*Weaving*—In wool, linen, cotton, jute, coir yarn, etc.

*Carpet and Rug-Making*—In wool, jute, etc.

*Mat-Making*—In wool, rubber, jute, coir fibre, leather, wire, rags, etc.

*Papercraft*—Including paper cutting and folding, toys, notepaper and envelope manufacture, etc.

*Basketry*—In cane, willow, raffia, rush, etc.

*Cementcraft*—Coloured and plain in the manufacture of roof and floor tiles, drain pipes, chimney flues and pots, flower pots, garden furniture, etc.

*Leathercraft*—In the manufacture of wallets, purses, bags, belts, cases, trunks, book-covers, including plain, tooled and coloured work, etc.

*Glove-Making*—Including chamois and lined gloves, garden gloves and hedgers, felt gloves, knitted gloves, etc.

*Brushcraft*—Manufacture of toothbrushes, clothes brushes, boot brushes, sweeping brushes, scrubbing brushes, hair brushes, etc.

*Toy-Making*—Including wooden toys, tin toys, soft toys in wool and felt, cardboard toys, etc.

*Hat-Making*—In paper, felt, straw, wool, etc.

*Beadcraft*—For the manufacture of necklaces, bracelets, screens, cork mat borders, etc.

*Nettingcraft*—For the manufacture of tennis nets, fishing nets, flower nets, billiard pockets, etc.

*Printing and Book-Binding and allied activities.*

*Wirecraft*—In the manufacture of mats, bracelets, kitchen utensils, wire-fencing, etc.

*Design and Painting*—Including general painting, Christmas cards, showcards, stage scenes, etc.

*Dyeing*—Of wool, jute, linen, cotton, coir yarn, including the manufacture of inks, paints, etc.

*Products from Waste Materials*—Including mats from old rubber tyres and scrap rubber, leather, tailors' clippings, rags, etc; manufacture of flock for cushions from the teasing of condemned clothes; engineers' cotton waste from condemned cotton materials, reclamation of solder from old tins; wooden toys from packing cases and waste timber, etc.

*Upholstering and ancillary operations.*

*Metal Work*—Including jewellery and enamelling.

*Wood Polishing*—Including french polishing, wax polishing and oil polishing.

*Stencilling*; *Batik*; *Barbola*; *Raffia-Work*; *Pottery*; *Plastic Modelling*; *Artificial Flower Work, etc.*

2. *Recreational:* This includes all forms of recreation, including social activities. It adds to the diversity and novelty of the treatment and provides a complete change from the handicraft side or work proper. It may be either (a) *active* or (b) *passive*, the latter including concerts, cinematograph or other entertainments, where the patient is merely a passive participant, the amusement being provided by others. Active recreational therapy is so designated, because the patient actively participates in the treatment and includes gymnastics, physical drill, calisthenics, music, dancing, indoor and outdoor games, picnics, country walks, featuring of plays and concerts, library activities, study circles, etc., and other social activities.

3. *Re-educational:* Re-educational Therapy, often referred to as Habit-Training, is a specialised form of occupational therapy, particularly applicable to the regressed type of mental case that has become 'wet and dirty' in habits. General habit-training is an important factor in the treatment of aments or mental defectives, but the re-educational form of the treatment is only suitable for regressed psychotics. It consists of a 24-hour balanced schedule of work, rest and play, which tends to restore lost or dormant habits, essential for proper social conduct and personal cleanliness. In addition to the inculcation of desirable habits, an improvement in the mental level is also achieved, which facilitates the gradation arrangement of both the craft and recreational elements of the treatment. The details of the therapy are elaborated fully in chapter nine.

Based on application, there are two broad divisions of the treatment, dealing with (1) Mental Disease and (2) Physical Disease and these are further classified according to the type of hospital concerned.

(1) Dealing with mental disease, the treatment will vary in certain details of organisation and application in the following hospitals:—(a) Mental Hospitals, (b) Mental Deficiency Institutions and (c) Epileptic Colonies. It is in mental hospitals, which deal with all forms of mental

ailments, that occupational therapy has reached the highest standard of perfection and application. Details of training courses give pride of place to the requirements of occupational therapy in mental nursing and practical training in a mental hospital is an essential qualification for all trained therapists. The mental hospital occupies the main outlet for advanced occupational treatment and, in a very singular way, exhibits all phases of the therapy, whether handicraft, recreational or re-educational. This is true, to some extent, also, in the case of mental defective institutions and epileptic colonies, which may be regarded as specialised types of mental hospitals, where the occupational work is graded to meet the respective needs of the patients in each case. In the case of mental deficients, the treatment must also be based on vocational lines to equip the higher grade types with the means of securing their own livelihood and, thus, returning them to the world as useful members of society.

(2) The treatment of physical disease also comes within the ambit of occupational therapy and its method of application is dependent on the type of disease or hospital in question. The range of hospitals now availing of occupational treatment is on the increase and among them may be cited the following: (a) General Hospitals; (b) Tubercular Sanatoria; (c) Children's Hospitals; (d) Convalescent Hospitals; (e) Orthopaedic Hospitals; (f) Correctional Institutions; (g) Orphanages; (h) Blind Asylums, etc. The method of treatment varies in all these types of hospitals and institutions; in the latter three, the vocational aspect is kept to the forefront. In all hospitals, active occupational treatment is definitely contraindicated in the acute stages of disease, especially when any degree of pyrexia is present. In general hospitals, a variety of conditions have to be dealt with and suitable occupational treatment prescribed. Cases requiring rather long periods of hospitalisation, such as heart cases, nephritics, general surgical cases, cases of chronic arthritis, peripheral neuritis and many others, as well as all conditions involving prolonged convalescence, must be prescribed for occupationally on the respective needs of each case. Bedside occupations have to be provided for, as well as a special centre suitably situated.

The organisation and development of occupational therapy in all these various hospitals and institutions, just mentioned, vary, to such an extent in each case, from standard psychiatric practice, that it is not possible, in a text-book of this kind, to cover, adequately, all the details associated with such specialised forms of the treatment. All are governed by the same primary principles already enunciated, though each demands special adaptation of the treatment to suit the requirements of each type. Modifications of the treatment, so elaborately developed in psychiatric hospitals, will be necessary to adapt it for use in dealing with physical diseases. The conditions to be encountered in a tubercular sanatorium will vary in many details and circumstances from those which prevail in an orthopaedic hospital and the latter will create problems, additional to those prescribed for in a general hospital. Children's hospitals, too, will make very special demands on an occupational therapy department, that will have to be dealt with in the light of modern principles of child psychology. All these should, accordingly, be covered in a special treatise or in a series of such texts.

In addition to classifying the hospitals, it will be necessary to classify the different types of patients met with in each hospital. Each case must be placed in a definite category to facilitate proper prescription and prevent negative results. The turbulent and noisy case must be considered apart from the quiet and demented case and special consideration must be given to the melancholic and suicidal type. In tuberculosis, the bed cases are given separate treatment from the ambulant types and both are graded off from the semi-ambulant patients, whose treatment occupies an intermediate position to the two former. The occupational treatment of orthopaedic conditions, involving muscle, bone and joint diseases, has to differentiate between the acute early stages of the disease from the later stages, when functional restoration is chiefly aimed at.

An analysis and classification of the various crafts and occupations, availed of, is also essential to secure the best results. The different occupations must be graded to suit the mental capacity of the demented, as well as the more intelligent type of patient. On the mental side, the different crafts are generally divided into two main classes, according as they are (1) sedative or (2) stimulative. The fatigue element in each craft will also have to be considered as well as the difficulty of performance or otherwise. They must be applied to maintain the patient's interest and avoid any tendency to discourage him. Likewise, the posture, required in the performance of each craft, is of the utmost importance on physical grounds. Faulty posture leads to early fatigue and increased eye strain, which may be further accentuated by arranging the work so that the patient may be facing the light. The importance of all these details points to the necessity for a proper classification and exhaustive analysis of the different handicrafts, which is dealt with later in the case of the three major crafts.

Consideration must also be given to the personnel of the occupational therapy department to secure due apportionment of the responsibilities of the staff concerned in the different phases of the treatment. The duties in each case must be fully defined to prevent overlapping and to co-ordinate the activities of all sections into an harmonious whole. Each unit must contribute its share and co-operate with the others in reaching the general therapeutic goal of the treatment. This is dealt with, in detail, in the next chapter.

4. *Commercial*: An additional section of an O.T. department, concerned, solely, with the economic, as distinct from the therapeutic aspect, must receive due consideration. Such consideration, however, must not over-ride the main therapeutic functions of the department. In the various general and other clinical hospitals, where the development and promotion of treatment is the primary object and always kept in the forefront, the financial and commercial administration of these hospitals is always based on proper, business-like methods and this viewpoint is maintained without, in any way, interfering with the therapeutic requirements. Likewise, in psychiatric hospitals, the functions and purpose of the O.T. department are in no way altered by the adoption of correct and sound economic procedures. The efficiency and success of the latter react most favourably on the standard

of results in the former.    Both are mutually interdependent, with the latter giving way to the former, whenever necessary.

Equipment and subsequent maintenance, as well as the continuous purchase of materials therefor, with resultant disposal and sale of the finished products, create a host of additional responsibilities for the chief occupational therapist and his deputies. These operations, involving such a huge amount of clerical and accountancy work and incidental interlocking with the pre-existing commercial activities of the hospital, make it necessary to discuss them at length. This is elaborated fully in chapter ten.

# CHAPTER V.

## DEVELOPMENT AND ORGANISATION

### ADMINISTRATIVE PERSONNEL

THE DEVELOPMENT and organisation of an occupational therapy department in a hospital will depend on the type of hospital and the number of patients requiring treatment. It is proposed to discuss the position in a mental hospital consisting of approximately 1,000 patients, male and female, and modifications may be substituted to meet the needs of other types of hospitals. We must consider (1) the administrative personnel, outlining the functions and status of each member and (2) the various units and sections of the department, explaining their relation to the staff and to each other.

With a view to securing the maximum benefits of occupational therapy, to embrace all its forms and to extend its scope, so as potentially to reach every patient in the hospital, it is essential to appoint an *Occupational Therapist* for each side of the hospital, with a *Chief Occupational Therapist.* The latter will be answerable to the *Medical Superintendent* for the working of all departments, both male and female. The occupational therapists will be, as it were, the liaison officers, acting as the connecting link between the detailed operation of the treatment and the *medical and lay officers of the hospital.* They will be assisted, in turn, by (1) *Technicians,* skilled in certain handicrafts; (2) *Nurses,* who may have some technical knowledge or secured certificates in occupational therapy and are styled *Occupational Nurses* and, lastly, (3) *Nurses* with nursing experience only. The position and inter-relation of all these are shown in the graph on the next page, *Fig.* 1:—*Page* 48, as well as their association with the members of the clerical and stores staff, concerned in the commercial or business aspect of the treatment.

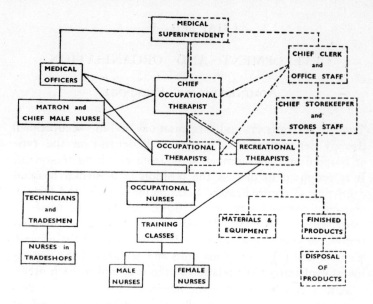

*Fig.* I

The above diagram, Fig. I, lists in schematical form, the various members of the mental hospital staff, who may be associated, directly or indirectly, with the administration of occupational therapy. The officers on the left half of the diagram, outlined in black, take part directly in the clinical development of the treatment, each in his or her respective section. The medical officers and senior nursing officers are associated in a supervisory capacity, in collaboration with the various occupational therapists, in directing the many different sections, which are in the charge of occupational nurses, technicians, etc.

The officers in the right half of the diagram, outlined in dotted surround, are concerned only with the commercial or business side of the treatment, in the same manner as their other duties are related to other phases of hospital administration. The clerical and stores staff collaborate with the medical superintendent and occupational therapists in the purchase of materials and equipment as well as in the disposal and sale of all O.T. products.

The detailed duties and role played by each officer listed are discussed as follows:—

*The Resident Medical Superintendent*, as chief executive officer of the hospital, responsible to his Committee or Board of Management for every phase of the hospital administration, must, as in all other sections, be in supreme control of the occupational therapy department. He must allocate and supervise the duties of each member of the staff concerned in the treatment and weld them all into a working whole. He must, as it were, assume the role of captain, directing, advising and controlling the activities of each member of his occupational therapy team. He must ensure that each member is in the correct place allotted to him and that all combine to secure the maximum team results. He will be supported by his medical officers, acting as vice-captains, and will give to each of them the responsibility of directing different sections of the treatment. He will direct and collaborate with the chief occupational therapist and the clerical and stores staff in the administrative and commercial details of the treatment. He will, likewise, supervise and consult with the medical staff and the occupational therapists on the different therapeutical problems that may arise and receive reports from all his officers on the progress of their respective sections.

He will, in fact, have to be conversant with every detail of the treatment and report fully each year on the progress of the department. It will be appreciated, therefore, that the medical superintendent's duties and responsibilities connected with occupational treatment are manifold and complex. They make administrative demands of a most unusual kind and call for special aptitudes and knowledge not usually associated with the qualifications of a medical superintendent. He must, accordingly, be versed, in a general manner, in both the theory and practice of the treatment. Unless he possesses a knowledge of the theory and principles involved, the primary and basic object of the department may be lost sight of and the therapeutic aspect will become enmeshed in the economic and commercial net of the administration. This will result in the establishment of a series of industrial occupations, subserving the financial interests of the hospital only and ignoring the primary therapeutic purpose.

The medical superintendent must be conversant with the organisation and practical application of the treatment in all its phases and ramifications in the special centres, trade-shops, wards, etc. While not requiring a skilled and technical knowledge of the various crafts, he must have a general and theoretical acquaintance with the procedures connected with each occupation. He must distinguish between the ward and bedside occupations, between the special trades and crafts and understand the comparative analysis of each. He must be in a position to advise on the number and variety of crafts and consider the introduction of any new occupations in the light of their therapeutic, nursing and commercial possibilities. He must have a thorough knowledge of the duties and functions of each member of the personnel of the occupational therapy staff and must act in a supervisory role in directing the entire department.

The duties of the *Medical Officers* will depend on their number and the size of the hospital. Where only two medical officers are available, one is allotted to the female section and the other to the male section and each collaborates with the chief occupational therapist and the respective occupational therapists in directing the work. Each completes the occupational prescription cards for his respective side and makes the necessary recommendations for treatment, outlining the main symptom-content and enumerating the aptitudes and idiosyncrasies in each individual case. In addition to receiving written reports, the progress of each case is followed and variations in treatment are discussed and recommended. Promotions and progress in each step of the treatment are observed and recorded and appropriate reports made to the medical superintendent.

All forms of the treatment must be supervised under the direction of each occupational therapist—occupational work in the reception wards, bedside occupations, the tradeshops, special craft centres, etc., recreational activities and re-educational programmes. Each medical officer must co-operate with the occupational therapists in the training of the nursing staff for the furtherance and proper development of the treatment. Theoretical lectures must be given in psychological medicine in relation to occupational therapy. Ward classes must be organised for practical training in the application of the various crafts, as well as for recreational and re-educational activities. Facilities must be provided and the nurses encouraged to acquire certificates in occupational therapy in order to secure the maximum development and success of the treatment.

The role played by each medical officer is, therefore, a most important one and the success of the scheme will be dependent on the interest displayed by them. Each medical officer must be grounded in the principles and practice of the treatment. He must collate the individual interests and aptitudes in each case with the intellectual and emotional tendencies in reaching the most suitable prescription. Special mental symptoms must be indicated for the guidance of the O.T. staff concerned and these must be considered in their relation to each particular craft in a complete analysis of the latter.

It will be noted, therefore, that the relationship of the medical officers to occupational therapy is a very close one. Their association is of a much more active type than might appear at first sight. They are responsible for introducing the patients to the treatment on prescription and are expected to follow up the progress of their cases in the various steps of the treatment. This entails visits to each occupational centre in addition to the ward activities and includes active supervision of the recreational facilities included under the treatment. Hence the medical officers, as in other forms of therapy, must make a definite study of all branches of the treatment to ensure that the primary principles underlying it are kept to the forefront.

In the case of hospitals where more than two medical officers are attached, further divisions of the treatment may be adopted to reduce the amount of responsibility and supervision in each case. Where three doctors are resident, one may assume charge of the special craft centres and tradeshops, the two other confining their activities to the occupational activities of the various wards. If a fourth doctor is available, he may be given supervision of the rec-reational and re-educational sections of the therapy and, similarly, the occupational activities in the wards on each side may be further divided to provide for supervision by additional medical staff. It can be readily appreciated that a large medical staff, with consequent reduction in their responsibilities and supervisory duties, will lead to a more efficient and detailed application of the therapy in all its branches.

*Occupational Therapists:* While in a small mental hospital, one occupational therapist, with the assistance of a number of technicians and occupational nurses, under the guidance and supervision of the medical staff, may successfully con-duct, for at least a period, an occupational therapy department, this is certainly not practicable in a hospital containing 1,000 patients. The extent of the work and organisation involved in the latter necessitates, not alone two occupational ther-apists, one on each side of the hospital, but, also, a chief occupational therapist.

*The Chief Occupational Therapist* will be responsible to the medical superintendent for the development and progress of the whole occupational department on both sides of the institution, including every phase and section of the treatment. While delegating immediate responsibility for the working details to her respective occupational ther-apists, she will act in a supervisory capacity under the direc-tion and authority of the medical superintendent and collab-orate with the various medical officers in the sections allotted to them. She will promote the initiation of any new sections or developments of the treatment as the necessity arises, and advise on the introduction of new crafts and occupations, both from their therapeutical and commercial standpoints.

Further to her supervisory duties mentioned, she will, under the guidance of the medical superintendent, assume control of the commercial and business side of the treatment. She will be responsible for the purchase of raw materials and equipment required and collaborate with the storekeeper in its distribution to the various sections. She will co-operate with the stores staff in the checking and receipt of the finished articles and will deal exclusively with their sale and disposal, whether to the hospital or to the public or outside concerns. She will assume full responsibility for the general records of the treatment, both therapeutic and commercial and supply all the statistical information required, writing up all the necessary ledgers and registers and making all necessary reports to the superintendent.

The duties of the occupational therapists, on each side of the hospital, will be confined purely to the therapeutic aspect of the treatment, excepting the completion of accounts or ledgers as directed by the chief occupational therapist. They will supervise the distribution of materials to the various sections in their respective sides, as well as the collection and transmission of the finished articles to the stores. As already pointed out, the occupational therapists will have to be officers trained and qualified in accordance with specially accepted standards. They will have to possess a detailed knowledge of the various crafts, both in theory and application, with special aptitude for instructing and teaching the nursing staff. They must be thoroughly acquainted with the technique and intricacies of each occupation, noting the therapeutic and commercial advantages. They must be able to apply the most advanced methods of imparting to their patients a working knowledge of all crafts. They will have acquired an appropriate knowledge of psychology and psychological medicine to enable them to interpret correctly the medical prescriptions passed on to them and so secure the best therapeutic results in each case. They will have received practical instruction in the different recreational and re-educational activities associated with the treatment and be in a position to supervise their introduction into the occupa-tional therapy programme.

It is presumed that female occupational therapists are generally appointed, though male therapists, where available, may also be employed. The functions in both the male and female sides of the hospital will be more or less identical, apart from adjustments, which the exigencies, appropriate to each side, demand. They will be responsible to the chief occupational therapist for the receipt of materials and equipment and the conversion of the materials into the finished products, and will have to complete the necessary ledgers and books giving these details. They will have to keep all the records denoting the progress of each individual case, as well as the progress of the department generally, giving occupation details of each section of the treatment under their supervision and submit these regularly to the medical staff concerned. They will have to consult and co-operate with the medical officer allotted to each section, discussing the results of treatment, both individually and collectively, introducing any recommended variations and alterations.

They will be responsible, in conjunction with the medical officers, for instructing the nursing staff in the theory and practice of occupational therapy, giving lectures at suitable hours and arranging practical classes in the wards and at the special occupational centres. As much of the success of the department will depend on the support and assistance of the associated nursing staff, this, in turn, will depend, to a large extent, on the success of the teaching methods adopted and the amount of attention and time given to the training of the staff. Too much stress, therefore, cannot be laid, especially in the initial stages, on the importance of suitable training facilities and the necessity for inculcating proper technique and sound therapeutic principles. Failure to do so, by the therapist, may inevitably lead to incorrect outlook on the part of the nurses and a faulty appreciation of the rationale of the treatment, economic and production objectives may thus become the sole guiding factor in the mind of each nurse, who may thus tend to regard their patients in terms of output units rather than in therapeutic units. Thus the whole object of the treatment may be defeated by the failure to ensure correct standards of training and proper grounding in the basic principles and objects of the therapy.

*Technicians:* These would include the skilled tradesmen, who are generally attached to the staff of mental hospitals, either in a temporary or permanent capacity, and also trained craftsmen with a practical knowledge of one or more handicraft of a specialised nature. The former would comprise the woodworker, shoemaker, painter, plasterer, mason, tailor, upholsterer, engineer, seamstress, etc. The tendency has been to regard these tradesmen from the utility viewpoint, whose chief purpose in the hospital is that of maintenance and to allocate to each of them a certain number of patients, based usually on their output capacity and the output requirements of each trade. Under a fully organised occupational therapy scheme, these tradesmen would be regarded as technicians instructing and advising the patients and staff in their charge, in their respective crafts and assuming charge of special occupational centres in their shops. They would, for occupational therapy purposes, be subject to the occupational therapists and their technical knowledge would be invaluable in solving the craft problems that arise in their own centres. They open up channels for developing the occupational needs of expanding departments and can be useful instructors in training the nursing staff, especially the occupational nurses, who may be described as O.T. nurses.

With the expansion of the department and the introduction of more advanced and specialised crafts, the necessity arises for the appointment of skilled craftsmen, who possess advanced knowledge of one or more of these crafts, such as printing and book-binding, weaving, metal work, basketry, tinsmithwork, etc. These would, thus, be available to assist and instruct the patients in the more difficult points encountered in the progress of these crafts, as well as to teach the members of the nursing staff associated with the treatment. Due to their lack of knowledge in the nursing of mental conditions and their inexperience of the therapeutic aspect of the work undertaken, they must, in the initial stages, be assisted by a nurse to the mutual advantage of each and the general good of the department.

*Nurses:* These will be divided into two classes, those with nursing experience only and those who possess, in addition, a knowledge of the occupations generally in use. The latter are styled *O.T. Nurses.* When establishing and developing the treatment, the occupational therapists will often be in a position to select, from the existing staff, a few nurses who have had some experience of handicrafts and are capable of instructing the patients in these. They will have a good deal of experience of mental nursing and must possess a mental nursing certificate. Their practical knowledge of the occupations must be supplemented from both theoretical and practical lectures delivered by the medical staff and the occupational therapists, stressing the therapeutic aspect of the work and the application of the treatment from that angle, in all its phases. In time, these O.T. nurses may be completely relieved of ward duties and take charge of different sections, as allotted by the occupational therapists, one or more to the handicrafts side, as well as to the recreational and re-educational sections. They may, also, be in a position to give practical instruction to the nurses who will be assisting them and should be ranked of equal standing to ward charge nurses.

The nurses, generally, must co-operate in the development of the treatment in the wards and various other sections of the hospital, if successful results are to be attained. They must help in the establishment of bedside and ward occupations and assist in their operation. They must carry out duties in the various centres and tradeshops and take an interest in the therapeutic and practical side of the work. They must join in the recreational activities promoted, including physical drill and calisthenics and co-operate in the habit-training programmes arranged for the regressed patients. They will receive suitable theoretical lectures from the medical officers and occupational therapists and will attend practical training classes arranged in both the wards and occupational centres. They should regard the application of the treatment as a change of work rather than added work and should enter into the spirit of the treatment, attaching to it the same significance and importance as to all other forms. They should not view it as an extra burden making extra nursing demands. They should feel that the more monotonous task of mere ward supervision is replaced by the more absorbing and interesting methods of occupational treatment.

A brief reference must be made here to the other non-medical or *Lay Officers* of the hospital and their relation to the occupational department. These include the Matron, Head Male Nurse, Clerk or head of the office staff, Head Storekeeper, Land Steward, etc. While the occupational therapists will not be responsible directly to the matron or head male nurse, the latter will be expected to co-operate and facilitate the smooth working of the details of the treatment in their respective sections. They must make suitable provision for the appropriate distribution of the staff and patients to the various centres and remove any obstacles that might tend to hamper the progress of the department. They must collaborate with the occupational therapists in dovetailing the different sections of the treatment into the general working routine of the hospital and thus accept it as a further commendable addition to the existing forms of treatment available.

The chief occupational therapist will confer with the *Chief Clerk* and the office staff in dealing with the large amount of clerical work involved in the purchase and sales side of the department. He will similarly supervise, with the stores staff, the checking and accounting associated with the purchase of materials and equipment and their distribution to the occupational sections, as well as the receipt of the finished articles and their disposal through sale to the hospital or otherwise. He will also be facilitated by the *Land Steward* and the *Engineer* in providing suitable occupations in their respective sections, as well as the heads of the laundry and kitchen and other utility departments.

In fact, every member of the staff must contribute towards the full development of the treatment as far as lies in his or her power and its success will be largely dependent on the volume of support accorded by the staff as a whole. There will scarcely be a single member of the staff, whose routine duties will not bring him or her in contact, in some way, large or small, with the occupational therapy department, when he or she will be called upon to make some positive contribution towards its development. Failure to co-operate will be a weakening of the link in the lengthy

therapeutic chain, which ramifies through the entire institution. All members of the staff, therefore, must give the
assistance and co-operation, commensurate with their responsibilities, in the organisation and development of the
treatment.

# CHAPTER VI.

## DEVELOPMENT AND ORGANISATION *(contd.)*

## SECTIONS AND UNITS

### HANDICRAFT SECTION

UNITS AND SECTIONS OF O.T. The three main sections of the treatment, as already stated, are (1) *Handicraft*, (2) *Recreational* and (3) *Re-educational* or *Habit-Training* and each will be composed of different units as charted on page 63 (Fig. 4). This diagram also shows, in dotted outline (4) *The Commercial Section* dealt with in chapter 9, which is a non-therapeutic section.

(1) *The Handicraft Section* consists of three main units, (a) *The Special Occupational Centre*, (b) *The Ward Occupational Activities* and (c) *The Utility Departments*.

(a) *The Special Occupational Centre* is the pavilion or building where the special and advanced crafts are organised and houses the main activities of the treatment. All the advanced and more technical occupations are put into operation here, excepting the work associated with the various tradeshops, where the special facilities already provided, including machinery and technical supervision, justify their non-inclusion in the former. The extent and size of the special occupational pavilion will be dependent on the number and type of crafts in general use and it would be impossible to plan a standard type of structure that would prove suitable for all hospitals. Many hospitals may possess some central building that might be adapted for the purpose. The rough sketch plan (Figs. 2 and 3 on pages 60, 61) should meet the needs of such a pavilion. It includes a central showroom and administrative offices, which cannot be adequately provided for in any other part of the institution and the necessity for which is an indication of the clerical, commercial and administrative responsibility entailed in a properly and fully developed occupational therapy department. It is only those, who are unaware of the extent of the latter, cannot understand the necessity for such a central occupational building.

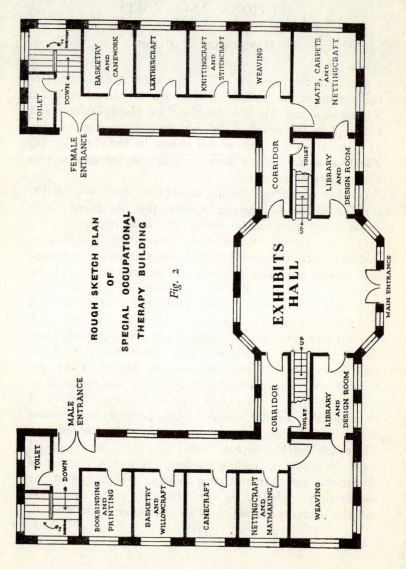

ROUGH SKETCH PLAN
OF
SPECIAL OCCUPATIONAL
THERAPY BUILDING

*Fig. 2*

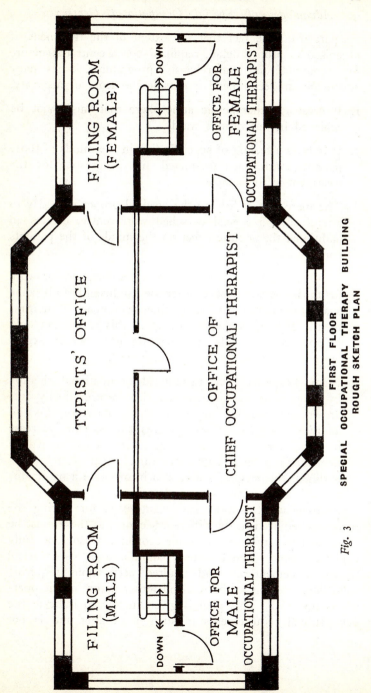

FILING ROOM
(FEMALE)

DOWN

OFFICE FOR FEMALE
OCCUPATIONAL THERAPIST

TYPISTS' OFFICE

OFFICE OF
CHIEF OCCUPATIONAL THERAPIST

FILING ROOM
(MALE)

DOWN

OFFICE FOR MALE
OCCUPATIONAL THERAPIST

*Fig.* 3

FIRST FLOOR
SPECIAL OCCUPATIONAL THERAPY BUILDING
ROUGH SKETCH PLAN

### *Advantages of Special Occupational Centre:*

Apart from the fact that the extent of the treatment, if organised in proper detail, requires such a central structure for a complete and comprehensive programme, it has many advantages to recommend it outside the score of necessity.

1. It creates a therapeutic atmosphere that might not be achieved in the various wards.

2. It imbues a feeling of specialisation in the minds of those patients, who have graduated and progressed for the treatment in this centre.

3. The mere fact of leaving the hospital proper each day to attend such a special detached work-centre, creates an additional therapeutic effect on the minds of the patients concerned.

4. It further tends to create a normal atmosphere of work for those cases that have progressed sufficiently to become susceptible to the socialising influence of an active environment. The psychological aspect of this factor can only be appreciated through the medium of a practical experience rather than by theoretical appeal.

5. Many hospitals have introduced occupational therapy by a series of ward expansions that have gradually outgrown the available space and the progressive effect of additional occupations, entailing as it does, a vast increase in administrative responsibilities, creates an immediate demand for such a central structure. In the sketch plans outlined, this structure may also incorporate a basement, as well as the two stories described.

The provision of a basement is suggested for storing the materials required in the different sections, as these must be purchased in large quantities for economic reasons, as fully explained later. The basement could also be used for all forms of cementcraft and kindred occupations requiring solid floors, owing to the wet and messy nature of the operations involved. This plan is given merely to indicate the occupational requirements in such a building and is not intended to dictate to architects, who may wish to arrange the plan and design to meet local conditions as the latter must be a determining factor in the final style of such a structure.

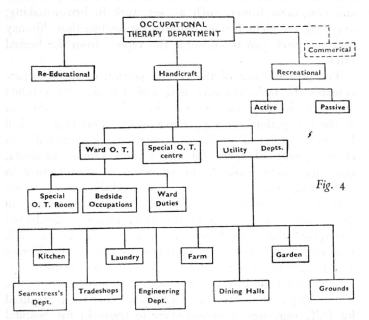

Fig. 4

The relative arrangement of the different crafts in the rooms provided must be based on the supervisory demands made by each occupation. The size of the rooms may also be proportioned in each case to meet the needs of each occupation, but there are certain essentials that must be insisted on even against the possible advice of the architect. The ceilings should never be less than 12 feet from the ground and should, if possible, be 14 feet. The question of lighting is of paramount importance and should be the maximum possible. This can be effected by the conversion of practically the entire external wall space of each room into long windows, reaching close to the ceiling and of the low-silled type. This arrangement must be insisted on even to the detriment of external architectural appearance and even with this limitation, architectural genius will find

suitable expression in other directions to ensure a pleasant
aesthetic effect. This increased window space will also
lend itself to proper ventilation, which must be specially
attended to in the case of those crafts, which create poisonous
and obnoxious fumes, such as, set work in brush-making,
dye-craft, etc. The former requires a special suction chimney
over the pitch pan to consume the vapour from the heated
pitch.

The ground floor of the central portion of the structure
contains the main entrance hall, which houses the exhibits
and gives to the inexperienced visitor his first introduction
to the occupational therapy department. This exhibits hall
has been designed of large proportions, intentionally, to
ensure plenty of space for the various sample products,
showing, where feasible, the processes of manufacture in
each case. The arrangement of the exhibits must be on
tasteful and attractive lines, such as to give the visitor an
instantaneous impression of the O.T. activities conducted
throughout the entire hospital. On either side of this hall,
with entrance therefrom in each case, is situated the library
and design room for male and female sides, respectively,
with special exits direct to the occupational therapy rooms.
These design rooms only house craft and other books required
for O.T. purposes, supplementary to those in the hospital
general library.

In the second floor of the central structure, in the corresponding space over the exhibits hall, is housed the chief
occupational therapist's room in the front portion and
an administrative or typist's office immediately behind.
On either side of the former and situated immediately overhead the library and design rooms, lie the offices, one for
each occupational therapist, with a direct entrance in each
case to the office of the chief occupational therapist.

(b) *The Ward O.T. Activities* are classified under three
heads, namely: (1) in the *Special O.T. Room*, (2) *Bedside
Occupations* and (3) *Ward Duties*.

(1) *The Special O.T. Room* may be Ward Dayroom, if
suitable, or some special room adjacent thereto, where suitable
crafts are introduced for those patients who, for mental

or physical reasons cannot be submitted for the treatment outside the ward. The treatment facilities in these cases will depend on the type of ward, whether it consists of recent, chronic, refractory, epileptic or the sick and infirm cases, or whether there is even still a more detailed classification based on the various mental disease types. In all cases, the crafts to be operated must be of such a nature as not, in the first instance, to necessitate any elaborate machinery or equipment that might, for various reasons, be contraindicated in any particular ward or, in the second place, to increase precautionary measures or supervision to an undesirable extent. They must further be of the simple, easily-grasped type and non-fatiguing, such as rag-teasing, mat-making, table looms, etc. For the chronic and mentally inaccessible cases, as well as the excited and destructive patients, there is no occupation that complies with the conditions mentioned to the same extent as rag-teasing. An endless amount of material is available, for this work, from the condemned stores, as fresh supplies are being constantly added from the routine condemnations of old and worn-out clothing. The teased material can be graded to make engineers' waste or even flock for cushions or filling material for soft toys. In the case of senile and chronically infirm patients and those convalescing from physical illnesses, netting can be introduced, whether on the circular or tennis net looms, as well as rope-plaiting and other lighter, non-monotonous occupations that tend to maintain the interest-element so essential for the treatment.

(2) *Bedside Occupations* have also been devised for those chronic cases who are more or less permanently confined to bed and also for those convalescing from acute illnesses and who, in both cases, are able to sit up in bed. There are no hospitals, mental, tubercular or general, that do not possess cases requiring bedside occupational treatment and the ward crafts mentioned can be adapted for bedside treatment purposes by the addition of a special frame or table astride the bed to hold the loom or other equipment or the materials in position, for operation by the patient, as he sits upright in bed. Convalescence, as we are aware,

is a very tedious and exacting period for both patient and medical attendant, especially when of a protracted nature, and there is nothing comparable with occupational therapy, even when confined to active or passive recreational activities, such as reading an interesting book or listening to a ward concert or attractive wireless programme. It is soothing to the patient and helps to tide him over this difficult period. It, in fact, tends to reduce the extent of the convalescent period—an important consideration, whether therapeutic or economic. The range of such occupations, even though limited in number, is yet sufficiently wide to ensure variety and is capable of further extension by a resourceful and ingenious therapist.

(3) A useful adjunct to the handicraft side of occupational therapy consists of the manifold *Ward Duties* that are routine in all hospitals and provide suitable occupation for a goodly number of patients in each ward for the greater part of each day. They consist of bedmaking, floorwashing and polishing, window cleaning and dusting, delph and ware washing, which varies in amount in each ward, brush-sweeping of all kinds and light repair work of one kind or another, transport of laundry to and from, as well as food when required, assisting the confused, restless and demented patients, who are incapable of attending to their entire toilet needs, etc. These ward duties are carried out under the different ward nurses, who generally supervise, but only rarely assist on those occasions when assistance becomes necessary. It is noteworthy the remarkable capacity displayed in training certain patients in each ward in this type of work, while there is sometimes a ready, though not very praiseworthy admission of failure, on the part of some of the nursing staff, in expending similar energy in other occupational therapy directions. This is demonstrated by the promotion of the more active of these ward duty patients to the special occupational therapy building and the subsequent speedy development in the ward of very competent substitutes.

(c) The last, but not the least important division of the handicraft section of the treatment is the *Utility Departments* of the hospital. These consist of the various upkeep and maintenance services of the hospital and are grouped, as follows:—

(1) *The Kitchen*, (2) *The Dining Halls*, (3) *The Laundry*, (4) *The Farm*, (5) *The Gardens*, (6) *The Grounds*, (7) *The Seamstress's Department*, (8) *The Tradeshops* and (9) *The Engineer's Department*. All these must be constituted as special occupational therapy sections, as the work attaching to most of them is of the skilled type. They are under the direction of individuals, each skilled and experienced in the work of his or her own particular department. These latter are classed as *Technicians*. These technicians, as already mentioned, must, in addition to their ordinary repair and maintenance work, be regarded as special craftworkers taking charge of special O.T. sections. They must advise and instruct the nurses and patients under their charge in the intricacies and difficulties experienced in their respective crafts and see that the maximum possible number of patients is submitted for treatment. They will, in this respect, be subject to the jurisdiction of the occupational therapists and will consult with them in all matters appertaining to the therapeutic side of their crafts.

(1) *The Kitchen*, as an occupational therapy department, will be in the charge of the cooking staff, who will supervise the nurses and patients allotted to their section and instruct them in the manifold duties associated with cooking and kitchencraft generally. The many processes through which food has to be submitted from its reception from the general stores to its final destination on the various dining hall tables, constitute a novel, interesting and skilled type of work that makes an immediate appeal to many patients. The resocialising effect of this type of work on most female patients and on many male patients gives the department a therapeutical importance that may, with difficulty, be equalled by the other utility sections. Here we find such diverse activities as mincing, washing, cutting, steaming, boiling, roasting, mashing, sifting, carting by hand or trolley, measuring, weighing, etc.

(2) *The Dining Halls* are an important utility department of the hospital, providing occupational treatment for a

large number of both male and female patients. The upkeep
and maintenance of the refectories involve a variety of
activities that are under the supervision of a skilled and
competent nurse. These include washing and cleaning the
ware and table utensils, the preparation of tables for the
different meals, as well as removal of waste food and the
general washing and cleaning of the halls. This work is,
in many hospitals, classed with kitchenwork generally, but,
owing to the nature and amount of the work concerned in
these sections, there is every justification for making them
separate, independent occupational sections.

(3) *The Laundry*, which is also under the control of a
special skilled staff, responsible to a head laundress, is much
akin to the kitchen in the diversity of the employment offered
and is capable of absorbing a large percentage of suitable
patients. Here, the steeping of clothes preparatory to washing,
preparation of laundry materials, assisting at the washing,
drying and ironing machines and hand ironing, call for
skill, attention and technical experience, which constitute
laundercraft, a highly therapeutic aid in occupational
treatment.

(4), (5) and (6) *The Farm, Garden and Grounds* are the
three sections under the skilled supervision of the farm
steward and his auxiliary staff of ploughmen, dairymen,
herdsmen, gardeners, etc. These, likewise, provide novel
and varying activities, which have the further commendable
advantage of open-air work. In providing for the special
aptitudes and wishes of the patients themselves, there is
here a special outlet, where indoor work of all kinds may be
objected to on many grounds, whether purely obsessional
or hygienic. Those with claustrophobiac tendencies may
persistently refuse to work in the occupational rooms until
their self-confidence is restored by special treatment. In
many hospitals where occupational therapy has not been
cultivated, these three sections have been mainly responsible
for absorbing the vast bulk of those patients who have been
returned as occupied.

(4) Work on *The Farm* is ever varying with the seasons
and can scarcely be equalled by any other section in the

amount and diversity of employment offered, some skilled, semi-skilled and unskilled. It includes the operation of the different machines in the cultivation of the land and the reaping of the harvest products, as well as the care and guidance of horses, the work concerned in the feeding and milking of the cattle, pig-rearing and fattening, poultry farming and the multiple manual labour activities associated with all forms of the agricultural industry.

A possible development in those hospitals with an exceedingly large acreage or with a large auxiliary farm at some distance from the hospital, is the establishment of a special farm colony or unit. This consists of a self-contained habitable pavilion, situated at some distance from the main hospital buildings, housing from 20 to 50 patients. It contains a suitable refectory, recreation rooms, dormitories and sleeping accommodation, kitchen, etc. Food is transported daily from the hospital and may be cooked in the pavilion. It is, in fact, a self-contained villa, with its own staff, both indoor and outdoor, and the enormous therapeutic effect of such a colony, with its socialising and stabilising influence, must constitute a very important branch of occupational treatment and one that makes a popular appeal to many recoverable cases.

(5) *The Gardens*, too, offer scope for outdoor activities of a very intriguing type to many patients, whose interest may be increased by the allocation of plots for individual cultivation. The attractiveness of the work is also enhanced by the range and diversity of activities. These include planting and cultivation of seeds and their subsequent transfer for flowering, fruit gardening and kitchen gardening. All these call for constant attention, with seasonal variations, that tend to increase interest in this craft.

(6) *The Grounds* under the direction of the farm steward, who allots supervision to one or more of his staff, require a certain number of patients for their care and maintenance and the amount of occupation available is dependent on the size of the latter and the type and extent of the lay-out. The avenues and approaches to the hospital require continuous attention, the lawns require cutting during season,

straightening the edges, etc. The gravel walks have to be
weeded and raked, as well as re-surfaced when necessary.
Hedges have to be clipped annually and receive general
attention. The trees, shrubs and plants, if not included in
the gardening section, also demand their quota of care.
The gatekeepers, if there is more than one hospital lodge
on the grounds, will be expected to increase the occupational
scope of this section in caring and beautifying the grounds
in the immediate vicinity of their lodges.

(7) *The Seamstress's Department*, which has always been
an important industrial section of all mental hospitals, will
easily lend itself to conversion into a very useful and practical
occupational centre. Like most of the industrial sections,
where therapeutic considerations have been lost sight of,
this department has been giving occupation to a limited
number of patients in many hospitals, with more concern
for output and production rather than for treatment and
recovery. As a consequence, the understaffing of this section,
both in the matter of technical and nursing supervision, as
well as patients, has created a condition of affairs where
the prevention of fatigue, as well as many other therapeutic
factors are subordinated to rushed output-results that are
opposed even to nursing principles. As a definite section of
the treatment, the seamstress should, as in all other departments, be assisted by occupational and other nurses and,
with extension of workrooms to meet requirements, should
provide treatment for treble the number of patients usually
employed, instead of forced work for a limited number.
The provision of the bulk of the clothing requirements of
the hospital, as well as the large amount of repair work, with
special machine equipment, supplemented by handwork, will
facilitate this suggested development. In addition to directing
this section, the seamstress will act in an advisory capacity
as technician with regard to all forms of stitchcraft, including
knitting. In fact, it may be feasible to make accommodation
for her department in the special O.T. building adjacent to
the rooms allotted for allied crafts and co-ordinate all these
latter under her technical supervision.

Finally, but not of least importance, we have (8) *The*

*Tradeshops* and (9) *The Engineering Department.* The points outlined in the previous paragraph apply with equal cogency to these two latter. Here there is ample scope, with increased accommodation made available, to treble or more the number of patients that can be submitted for occupational treatment in both sections. There is a regrettable tendency among the tradesmen to ignore the two-fold purpose of their employment and only to employ the minimum of patients that will not unduly add to their supervisory duties. Their primary purpose is to treat the maximum possible number of patients through the medium of their respective trades and, secondly, in this manner, to meet the repair and maintenance needs of the hospital. As shop accommodation is already in existence, with full and complete equipment for each trade, it is not usual to include provision for these sections in the special occupational therapy building, but there can be no objection to the suggestion if ample and properly equipped rooms are made available in each case.

*The Carpenter's Shop* should provide the nucleus of a large wood-working section, as the expansive possibilities of this craft are innumerable. It is even possible to develop many sub-sections of this, notably the manufacture of wooden toys, furniture, wood-turning and boring for brush stocks, etc. This is covered in much detail in the analysis of Wood-craft in a later chapter.

*The Painter's Shop* must also be of ample proportions to allow for the increased work in the painting and finishing of wooden toys and other products of the carpenter's section. As well as the painting, enamelling and varnishing of the different articles, provision must also be made for staining and polishing the products and with the different types of polishing that may be put in operation, it will be necessary to enlarge this shop to proper proportions or erect a suitable adjunct to provide for the additional work outlined.

*The Shoemaker's Shop*, in addition to providing for the boot needs of the entire hospital, will require a large number of patients for ordinary boot repairs. A good deal of the work will be skilled, but there will be some occupation available of a semi-skilled type, such as staining and polishing the shoes and the easier forms of patchwork, which are quite easily taught to many patients. The author has had experience in the case of a patient, who expressed a desire to work at the shoemaking trade and become quite proficient, even in the skilled side of the craft, after a period.

The work attaching to *The Plasterer's Shop* opens up further channels for employment by the development of cementcraft, which is associated with the plastering trade. The manufacture of roof tiles and floor tiles, both in colours, as well as drain pipes, chimney and flue pots and fence posts and garden furniture, demonstrates the flexibility of this craft and the large number of patients that may be so occupied, both in the preparation of materials and actual manufacture of the products.

*The Tailor's Department* corresponds, more or less, with the Seamstress's section on the female side and both are concerned with the clothing requirements of the hospital and the repair work incidental thereto. Here all the patients' suitings are completed from tweeds woven in the special O.T. centre and the section is capable of giving employment to a large number of patients. As far as men are concerned, it is more or less a skilled form of employment, but there is no reason why those, who express a desire to avail of this type of work, may not be given the necessary accommodation if suitable otherwise.

*The Baker's Department, The Mason's Section, The Upholsterer's Shop* and *The Stoker's Department* are other long-established sections in mental hospitals that can be treated as special occupational centres, giving suitable employment in certain cases recommended for these crafts and thus add to the very versatile nature of occupational treatment for mental cases.

(9) *The Engineering Department* opens up another very skilled type of work under the control of the chief engineer and a skilled auxiliary staff. These are responsible for the upkeep, repair and entire functioning of the different machines and engines situated in various parts of the hospital, as well as the repair and maintenance of the plumbing and heating systems, including the water supply and drainage systems.

The enormous amount of work involved in this department, mostly of a skilled type, makes it necessary to secure a good deal of assistance, which can absorb a large number of patients, both skilled and unskilled. The amount of iron-work undertaken and the provision of a forge, with lathes and other suitable machinery, suggest the possibility of developing a metal-craft section under a special occupational nurse with the engineer and staff acting as technicians for advice and assistance. This would increase the occupational possibilities of this section and give opportunity for providing the hospital with many costly metal products that have normally to be purchased from outside sources.

There are other departments in the hospital where occupational treatment is availed of on a small scale, but the number of patients dealt with in each case may not be sufficient to justify constituting them as special sections. These latter would include the offices, hall porter's department, stores, etc.

# CHAPTER VII.

## SECTIONS AND UNITS (*Contd.*)

### RECREATIONAL SECTION

### GENERAL ANALYSIS

A PROPERLY PLANNED PROGRAMME in a fully developed occupational therapy department must consist of a balanced arrangement of work, exercise and rest. Suitable provision having been made for sleep, the waking hours must be divided between work and exercise with appropriate intervals of rest, apart from meal times. In other words, recreational activities must find equal place with handicraft work in any well-balanced form of occupational treatment. Just as amusement, exercise and relaxation from the toils of the day are an essential feature of normal, healthy life, likewise, a proportionate distribution of work and amusement must be effected in the daily programme of the occupational treatment of the mentally and physically ill.

This section of the treatment is known as *Recreational Therapy* or *Diversional Therapy* and consists of both physical training and recreation, the former including gymnastics and calisthenics and the latter covering all forms of amusement and diversion, ranging from games, walks, music, dancing, concerts, dramatics, athletics, to active and passive bibliotherapy. Many authorities also incorporate in this section, the numerous hobbies that are of practical application such as gardening (personal plot development only), photography, caring birds and animals, philately, etc. These, however, do not run counter to similar activities in the handicraft section, as the latter are associated with productive results and not in vogue solely for diversional reasons. In other words, they have an utilitarian aspect that is absent

74

from purely recreational hobbies. This differentiation, however, does not alter the close connection, almost to overlapping, of the handicraft and recreational sections, as the element of occupation is a principle common to both, with the utilitarian and diversional aspects predominating respectively in each. Apart from this, the time-table and location of both departments, as well as the personnel and type of patients receiving treatment in each, have justified the constitution of both as separate sections of the occupational therapy department.

Likewise, it will be noted that physical training, included in this section, is an important feature of the rehabilitation programme of the special section forming the re-educational side of the treatment, covered in chapter 9. As this latter section deals with the reintegration of regressed psychotics by means of a special habit-training programme, it has resolved itself into a very specialised section of physical training and has, in fact, somewhat of a kindergarten outlook in acting as a training ground for promotion to the more advanced sections of the treatment. Physical training, including gymnastics and calisthenics, has a much wider application in the treatment of mental disease than for use in the case of normal, healthy people. Hall gives the following four aims of calisthenic exercise for normals:

1. To do everything physically possible for the body as a mechanism producing postures and attitudes never called for in life. This is the doctrine of multiform physical activity propounded by Jahn and further developed by Spiess.
2. Increased volitional control by practising these new movements, which stimulate conscious control rather than purely reflex activity.
3. Economic postures and movements.
4. Symmetry and correct proportions.

In this latter respect, physical training is concerned with purely bodily development. In dealing with mental disease, while these physical advantages are not to be minimised, their socialising and stabilising effect is of paramount importance. In promoting the reintegration of the psychotic, physical training influences the social maladjustment present and inducts the patient into a more acceptable social standard. The physical element of the treatment is definitely secondary to the psychical element.

Physical training must be distinguished from physical therapy, known as Physiotherapy. This has been defined as the treament of disease by means of the physical, chemical and other properties of heat, light, water, electricity, massage and exercise. It includes various subdivisions known as Hydrotherapy, Electrotherapy, Heliotherapy, Massage, etc. It is mostly a passive type of therapy and does not require the active co-operation of the patient during the period of treatment. Just as in the various forms of physiotherapy, definite results are achieved also by means of physical training and recreational activities. These are grouped under the following two heads: (1) *Physical* and (2) *Mental* or *Psychological.*

(1) Physical training and recreations of all kinds have a splendid tonic effect on the general musculature of the body, assisting in building up bodily tissues and restoring normal and correct posture. The muscular inactivity associated with disease, both mental and physical, must have a very deleterious and toxic effect generally and may result in constipation and other functional troubles. The muscular movements associated with the active type of recreational therapy play an important part in preventing such disturbances of function, as well as promoting general health.

Organically, the stimulation of respiration and circulation, by active body movements, must be beneficial to the well-being of all the vital organs. Digestion is thus promoted indirectly as well as reacting under the direct influence of the treatment. Disordered elimination of waste and toxic products is increased. In fact, all the vital and general organs of the body are stimulated, both directly and indirectly, to more healthy and active functioning.

In addition to the healthy development of the musculature and stimulation of various organs of the body, the general physical health is also benefited. There is developed a tendency to a better and more natural appetite. Insomnia, which is a troublesome feature of both convalescence and disease, is beneficially influenced and disturbed sleep is restored to a more normal health level.

These constitute the physical advantages of a recreational therapy régime and, while they may be accepted as the motivating principles of physical culture for normals, it must be borne in mind that the mental reactions to the treatment are the basic considerations. They are the most important guide as to its success as a therapeutic measure.

(2) On the *mental* or *physical* side, the general advantages of occupational therapy, outlined previously, apply with equal cogency here. Although the element of occupation may be common to both the recreational and handicraft side of the treatment and identical mental reactions may be created by both, there are special psychological results attained that are exclusive to each type.

(1) The chief and most important effect of recreational therapy is the tendency to promote resocialisation. Most psychotics and psychoneurotics come under notice because of their social maladjustments. Apropos of this, Bleuler states that:—

'So far as the concept of insanity has become at all practicable, it rests not upon medical or psychological criteria but on the idea of social incapacity.'

The socialisation of the patient becomes increasingly difficult owing to his inaccessibility through ordinary channels. Even persuasion and appeal may fail to make positive headway and approach in the initial stages may be possible only through the play instinct in order to establish contact. It is remarkable how many negativistic and resistive patients will respond by automatically returning a ball which is thrown to them. This instinctive act, uninfluenced by thought or judgment, or mental effort of any kind, is the first step towards resocialisation. This method of externalisation and resocialisation of the individual through recreational means is often the only method of approach in such types. It substitutes extroversion for introversion, turning the patient's mind from self to reality, from phantasy to fact.

(2) It promotes desirable interests, some of which may

have been repressed and are roused from dormancy to activity through graded recreation. New interests are also created, but the revival of dormant interests tends more towards the reintegration of the individual from physical to higher levels.

(3) It restores self-reliance, which appears to be undermined in the vast majority of psychotics. The patient's confidence in his own ability has been replaced by feelings of distrust and even fear and these emotions, which dominate consciousness, are best attacked by recreational means. Group activities create environmental conditions, which inspire self-trust and help to restore the healthy ambitions, which have become submerged by the psychosis.

(4) It resuscitates the normal response habits which have become confused or lost through regression and disintegration. Normal activity arises from a sensory stimulus, with physical response accompanied by a corresponding emotional response. The primary and simplest response is to food, while the secondary response, more important from the recreational point of view, is to physical activity. The latter, though hidden, may be brought to light by introducing the correct stimuli to restore these lost responses through some game, music or other recreational activity.

Most stimuli act through visual, auditory or kinaesthetic channels, that is, through sight, hearing or touch sensations or combinations of these. It is through these means, mostly, that we orientate ourselves with our surroundings and the failure of normal response to external stimuli constitutes the basic inactivity in psychotic disease. To replace the latter by healthy, physical activity is the object of recreational therapy and this is effected in an instinctive way, when direct appeal and persuasion may fail hopelessly. The imitative instinct, which is so prominent in children, can be readily roused, even in the most regressed type of patient and this becomes a potent factor in inducing the latter to respond to sensory stimuli. The majority of patients respond most readily to sensory stimuli of the visual type and will repeat movements performed in their presence, whether of the individual or group type. Others, who will not so react, may be influenced by verbal stimuli or by kinaesthetic sensations and can thus be inducted into recreational therapy, when handicraft therapy may be refused. In this way, it may be possible to overcome the hopelessness in combating the katatonic attitudes of negativism, stereotypy, 'flexibilitas cerea,' resistiveness, etc.

*Recreational Therapy* is broadly divided into two types—(1) *Active* and (2) *Passive*. The former is again subdivided into (a) *Intellectual* or (b) *Physical* and the passive type into (a) *Intellectual* and (b) *Sensory*. The active-intellectual and active-physical types may be further subdivided into (a) *Simplex* and (b) *Complex*. This classification for reasons of clarity has been charted on the next page. The division into active and passive has been based on the patient's attitude to the administration of the treatment. The therapy is of the active type when the patient participates actively in the recreation or other activities provided and is not a mere spectator or passive recipient of the treatment, as when listening to a concert or wireless programme, where others provide the therapeutic diversion. Examples of the active type are shown in athletics and various outdoor and indoor games, when the patient concerned is an active participant in them. The *passive* type of recreation is further divided into sensory and intellectual, but, it is sometimes difficult to observe the distinction, as there are mixed types, composed of both intellectual and sensory elements. In both cases, as stated, the patient is merely the passive recipient of entertainment provided by others and is described as sensory when it operates mainly through the bodily senses, mostly of sight and hearing. It is of the intellectual type when mental processes, mostly emotional, are the important feature, such as occurs when a member of a group listens to a lecture, reading, discourse or play. It is difficult to give an example of a pure sensory type, as intellectual elements are generally associated with all sense functioning—otherwise, it would be practically worthless as a therapeutic aid. The nearest to fulfilling the requirements outlined would appear to be listening to music provided by others, but, even here, the results desired can be reached only through the emotional element aroused and its consequent general effect.

The *active types* are again subdivided into intellectual and physical, according as the major degree of energy expended is of the intellectual or physical type. Examples of the former are participation in card or chess games, where the mind or intellect is mostly at work and the physical effort is almost negligible, resolving itself merely into pushing the chessmen or dealing and throwing the cards. The physical type would include the outdoor sports, swimming, football, running, jumping, etc., where the major portion of the activity is purely bodily. The active types, both intellectual and physical, are further sub-divided into simple and complex. The active physical types are designated as simple and active when the movements are of the single repetitive type, of easy comprehension and requiring the minimum of physical effort. An example of the latter would be a simple arm exercise involving a repetition of one single movement. Likewise, an example of the intellectual type would be a simple card game, where the intellectual effort concerned is so limited as to be almost absent, such as in 'beggar my neighbour.'

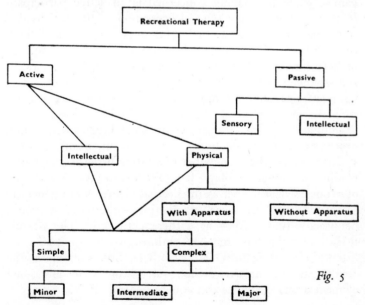

*Fig. 5*

*Complex active recreation of the intellectual type* is of such a nature as to bring into play a number of intellectual processes, involving memory, imagination, judgment and association of ideas. All these are brought to bear on the intricate problems that arise in a close, well-contested game of chess or on an intriguing hand of cards at a contract bridge table. The number and quality of intellectual processes at work in these instances are of such a complex nature that they must be distinguished from simple acts of intellection associated with minor intellectual forms of recreational therapy.

*Physical recreation of the active type* is designated as complex when it involves a medley and variety of movements, confined solely to the body musculature or in conjunction with special apparatus. Examples of the latter requiring special equipment would be skating, fencing, skiing and a medley race, composed of running, cycling, walking, hurdling, etc. Active complex recreation confined to unaided bodily movements would be exemplified in swimming, acrobatics, advanced drilling movements, etc. These fine-drawn distinctions may be somewhat arbitrary in a number of cases, when it may be difficult to avoid some overlapping, but such a grading and classification is a necessity when it is realised that there are so many different types of cases submitted for treatment depicting even many grades in the same disease. There must, in any case, be a gradation or stepping-stone arrangement in the application of this section of the treatment, as well as in the handicraft and other sections, and this can only be effected by such an exhaustive analysis of the recreational facilities available.

This comparative analysis in recreational as well as in handicraft therapeutics facilitates prescriptions in each individual case and assists the recreational therapist in the proper application of the treatment, whether of the individual or group type. It is absolutely essential to recognise at least the division of activities into simple and complex and it should be possible, in addition to the further subdivision of the complex type given above, to distinguish various grades of complexity with a view to establishing a definite gradation of activities from the lowest to the highest complex type. Subject to an accurate graphing of activities in grades of complexity, one must distinguish at least three broad grades, namely, (1) minor complex, (2) intermediate complex and (3) major complex. The minor complex type would be exemplified in calisthenics involving a repetition of two or three different movements, skiing, running, high jumping and elementary diving, while more advanced diving, hurdling, simple ballroom dancing, handball and calisthenics with a repetition of a variety of movements, would be classified as intermediate complex. Major complex activities would feature the most highly skilled and varied movements without the repetitive restrictions of the more simple complex type. These would consist of the more skilled and scientific games, such as tennis, advanced acrobatics, advanced gymnastics and calisthenics and intricate folk and ballroom dances, etc. The difference between gymnastics and calisthenics is recognised by the presence of apparatus to assist the bodily movements in the former and the complete absence of any mechanical assistance in the performance of the bodily movements in the latter. In the former, recourse is had to dumb-bells, clubs, parallel-bars, etc.

All diversional activities, therefore, must fall under one of these four heads, ranging from the simple to the major complex type and this gradation, associated with a suitable classification of the patients, recognising the individual as well as the group needs, is essential. An analysis and classification of the mental states of those submitted for treatment will be discussed in full in later chapters.

Mitchell and Mason have evolved the detailed classification of recreational activities, which is reproduced on page 83. The only objection that may be advanced to this list is the non-inclusion of gymnastics and calisthenics, whose omission may be due to their not being regarded as a play activity. Their importance, however, as a form of recreation and re-education has given them pride of place in these two O.T. sections. The list, also, would appear to regard the handicraft side of occupational therapy as a subdivision of play activity, while, as a treatment factor, handicraft work is accepted as being the primary and chief section, with recreational therapy considered as an important though necessary adjunct.

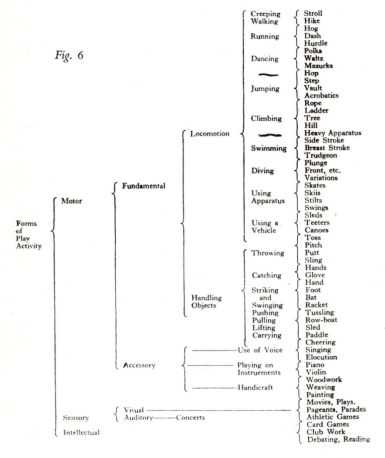

*Fig.* 6

Another classification of activities, as to form, has also been elaborated by Mitchell and Mason, as follows:—

'A.  Contests, between individuals and groups.

B.  Goal games such as hide and seek.

C.  Team games such as baseball.

D.  Combats such as wrestling.

E.  Hunting play such as trapping, angling, shooting or spearing.

F.  Curiosity play such as puzzle solving.

G.  Creative play such as art and craft work.

H.  Vicarious play such as looking at motion pictures.

I.  Imitative play such as following the leader in a folk dance.

J.  Acquisitive play such as collecting stamps.

K.  Social play such as impromptu party games.

L.  Aesthetic play such as clay modelling and painting.'

This classification repeats the objection mentioned above, in treating art and craft work as a form of play. There are many other classifications of recreational activities based on many different considerations, among which may be cited (1) individual and group activities, (2) indoor and outdoor and (3) formal and informal exercises.

(1) Arrangements must be made for *Individual and Group Activities* in the treatment. Following correct estimation of the volitional, emotional and intellectual capacities of a patient, individual treatment may be prescribed, where group treatment may be contraindicated. Administrative demands, however, will reduce such cases to the minimum number and promotion to group treatment must be aimed at in the final treatment of these types.

(2) From the point of view of adaptability and further to provide an essential novelty and variation, activities must be of both the *Indoor and Outdoor type*. This will heighten interest and encourage and maintain the attention so necessary for success, but, when possible, recreational activities should be mainly outdoor.

(3) *Formal Exercises* are those classed as educational and concerned with the correction of faulty postures and the promotion of proper function. They include corrective calisthenics, massage and other forms of physiotherapy. *Informal Exercises*, on the other hand, are of a purely social nature and consist of active games of all types, including athletics proper.

# CHAPTER VIII.

## SECTIONS AND UNITS (*contd.*)

### RECREATIONAL THERAPY SECTION

#### SPECIAL ANALYSIS

FOLLOWING the preceding general analysis of recreational activities, it is now necessary to discuss each individual recreation, particularly with regard to its development and organisation. An exhaustive, individual analysis is not possible within the limitations of a general textbook of occupational therapy such as this. The following list of recreational and diversional activities is not meant to be exhaustive, as local conditions and an ingenious therapist will add considerably to the list and there should be no limitations to the diversional development of the treatment:— dancing, calisthenics and gymnastics, outdoor games and athletics, indoor games, musical entertainments, cinema shows, dramatic performances, all forms of bibliotherapy, lectures, social entertainments, walks and hikes, motor and coach drives, sight-seeing excursions, seaside visits, hobbies, etc. There are many other activities not listed, but they are included as subdivisions of certain of the above recreations and will be discussed under the latter as they arise.

(1) *Dancing* is one of the oldest forms of recreational therapy and one that has found a place in the organised recreation of all mental hospitals, practically since their inception. It has a tremendous socialising effect and tends to reawaken dormant healthy interests even in regressed patients. As a form of entertainment, it can be of the passive as well as the active type; for many patients receive therapeutic benefit as spectators and enjoy both the music and the dancing. In this way, the range of the treatment is increased to reach a large percentage of patients. It likewise lends itself to both individual and group activity and has a versatility of expression and execution so important as a therapeutic measure. Varieties consist of ballroom, folk,

classical, clog, step and tap, and character dancing. Ballroom
dancing, including round dances, waltzes and foxtrots, etc.,
have, with folk dancing, the widest practical application
and are most in demand. Of the two, folk dancing is generally
regarded as exerting the greater therapeutic effect. They
are best known to the majority and are easily executed and
their entertainment value is not affected by absence of
proficiency or detailed knowledge of the component figures.
They are, in addition, of a more health-giving and energetic
quality, so necessary for certain types, and further, which
is probably the most important point, they are of a much
simpler rhythmic character than most other forms of dancing.

(2) *Calisthenics and Gymnastics* comprise formal exercises
that require to be specially adapted to meet the therapeutic
demands of a recreational therapy scheme. Of the two,
calisthenics, not requiring the aid of apparatus or special
equipment, is more in vogue. It permits of a series of graded
movements, from the very simplest single-repetitive type
to a series of maximum complexity. They, accordingly,
admit of grading to suit the most regressed dement at the
bottom of the scale and at the other end the most intellectual
psychoneurotic on point of recovery. They are suited for
individual and group application, with possibilities for
socialisation that render them indispensable in any comprehensive and well-balanced recreational programme. It
is urged, and with reason, that calisthenics of the command
and response type should be replaced by the more rhythmical
type, where waltz time should be substituted for march
time and fast jerky movements by the slower and more
rhythmical ones. The use of music for rhythm purposes
is strongly recommended, but should not enter so prominently into the picture as to cause distraction of attention;
it should be of the quiet background type, merely to indicate
the time and rhythm of the movements.

(3) *Outdoor Games and Athletics* open up a very wide field
for the application of recreational treatment of both the
active and passive type. Many patients who will not participate actively in the various games and sports will enjoy
looking at them, but the active side should reach the greatest

number of patients possible, as the maximum mental and physical benefits are derived therefrom. There is an inexhaustible list of outdoor games and sports, the vast majority of which are of practical application for therapeutic purposes and these admit of grading to suit the most deteriorated as well as the more intelligent patients. It must be remembered that the higher the degree of complexity and skill in any particular game, the greater is the tendency towards resocialisation. Further, the gradual promotion from the simpler to the more complex forms of recreation is an index of the success of the treatment in any individual case or group of cases.

Chief among outdoor games and constituting the vast majority of the latter, are ball games of all types, whether a ball is used exclusively or in conjunction with additional apparatus. They are, accordingly, placed first among outdoor activities as they are adaptable for accurate grading as to complexity and the therapeutic and other necessary values of any individual ball game are easily assessed. They range from the very simplest types, such as toss ball, pass ball, circle ball and bounce ball to the more complex games of football, handball, baseball, tennis, golf, etc. As with all outdoor games, they may be classified as individual or team games, where the competitive element based on scoring results is introduced.

There are many other games and sporting athletics proper, distinct from ball games, that are adaptable for recreational therapy purposes and possessing similar treatment values. Likewise, some of them require no special apparatus, such as swimming and diving, while others utilise special equipment to assist in the execution of the movements concerned, such as roller-skating, skiing, etc. They, too, admit of suitable grading with regard to the simplicity or complexity of the movements associated with each sport and are adaptable for individual or team application, as required.

*Athletics proper* also occupy a prominent position in recreational treatment programmes and one or more special days should be allotted for this purpose. This should be one of the special days set aside exclusively, as a gala day, when all other occupational therapy activities should be suspended and the entire hospital population participates in an active or passive capacity, as far as practicable. The programme should consist of running, jumping, weight-throwing, hurdling, tug-of-war contests and relay races, with the inclusion of novelty events, such as wheelbarrow races, obstacle races, egg and spoon races, sack races, etc. The hospital or other band should be present to play appropriate music during the progress of the sports. Suitable prizes or awards should be presented to the winners of the different events, as this completes the realism of the programme and contributes to the general socialising effect of the entire day.

*Team Games* should be encouraged so as to provide healthy competition among different sections of the hospital and these should act as trials for selection of teams, to represent the hospital, in the different forms of sport, in outside competitions. This latter arrangement, creating external contacts during hospitalisation, augments the therapeutic element of socialisation, which characterises all active recreational operations. It assists in inspiring the self-confidence so desirable for those patients who are convalescing for return to their former environment. The knowledge that their physical capacity is approximating normal standards of performance, creates desirable social and mental trends that tend to restore more normal thinking and conduct and thus hasten convalescence and recovery.

(4) *Indoor Games* are no whit less important than outdoor activities and help to balance the recreational programme as affected by both time and weather conditions. The restrictions imposed by shorter winter days and the vagaries of the weather in all seasons, must be met with the substitution of suitable indoor recreation for all outdoor activities. This requires the elaboration of a complete range of indoor games and other amusements to meet these conditions, in addition to the standard arrangement for daily indoor recreation. As with outdoor sports, there is no limit to the number and type of indoor games that may be found suitable for recreational treatment purposes. Heading the list are card

games of all kinds from the most elementary kindergarten type, such as 'donkey' and 'begger my neighbour' to whist and contract bridge. Card games are easily taught and while proficiency in play may only be within the compass of some more experienced patients, the amusement and emotional benefit to be derived will reach every patient capable of interpreting the relative values of the playing cards. Whist would appear to stand out as the most versatile game, being adaptable for four players or groups of four in the progressive variety. A playing knowledge of the game being easily acquired, it would lend itself to the organisation of whist drives on both a small and large scale. Small drives could be organised in any individual ward each evening, or at least weekly, while a central drive should be a regular monthly feature and of the mixed type, where the male and female patients and nursing staffs of both sides could participate. If conditions permit of it in any particular hospital, similar bridge drives might be arranged. These drives should be organised on similar lines, even to the smallest detail, to those arranged outside for normals. This inside duplication of normal conditions has an important bearing in influencing the correct emotional response for those who have been accustomed to participate in such social activities. It must in this way revive dormant social interests that have a definite influence on the stabilisation and socialisation of conduct.

There is a variety of indoor games, in addition to card games, that makes an appeal, where the latter fail to do so for many reasons. Among these may be cited chess, draughts, billiards, table tennis, quoits, dominoes and a host of others that are subject to current popularity. Most of these and especially billiards, form the basis for the organisation of tournaments on a large scale. The monotony of participating in individual contests is relieved by the widening of interests in a series of tournament games and increased numbers benefit from the passive recreation afforded. The element of chance as distinct from skill in many of these indoor games, has a widening effect in their application, and renders them suitable for the more regressed type of patients.

(5) *Musical Entertainments*, whether indoor or outdoor, provide active and passive recreational treatment of a wide and exceptionally comprehensive range. These include concerts, whether organised from within or without the hospital, musical wireless programmes, group or community singing, band promenades and musical cinema shows. Although the actual patient performers are receiving active recreational treatment, the therapeutic effect is secured mostly in a passive way, and in this manner reaches a large number, with little organisation and cost. The power and influence of suitable music has been recognised for normals from time immemorial and much has been written in its praise in every country. The genius of composers has been given to the world in the universal language of music, which is translated in an individual way that explains its universality. It reacts on the individual through the emotional feelings aroused and promotes healthy and desirable moods. It must, to a large extent, exert similar influences in cases of abnormalcy and must thus be regarded as of vast importance. It has the effect, when other means may fail, of holding the patient's attention and is often the only way to penetrate the curtain of inaccessibility that covers the most regressed type. Music, too, has a very favourable influence on the general atmosphere of the hospital. The atmosphere or composite environmental attitude of the patient population is nothing more than the 'emotional tone of the collective personality' of the hospital itself. Music, in an inimitable way, helps to convert an unfavourable atmosphere into one that is more infectiously cheerful and brighter. It radiates a happiness and serenity that endures beyond the actual rendering and gives a much needed and appreciated enjoyment to its performers and listeners.

*The Active Side of Musical Entertainments* has greater therapeutic possibilities than the passive type. In addition to the emotional elements mentioned, it provides intellectual stimulation of a therapeutic type in the interpretation and performance of the musical score. It creates an outlet for emotional flow and the dissipation of conflict, arising from repressed impulses. Healthy disciplinary trends are also aroused from the influence of group effort, which replaces undesirable autistic activities and thus provides an immediate opening into the road leading towards the normal mental goal. The performer, too, develops a very beneficial sense of emotional satisfaction from the feeling that he is contributing towards the entertainment of his listeners. Apart from community or group singing, however, musical entertainment of the active type has the great drawback of restricted application as it can only reach a limited number of performers.

*As a passive form of treatment, Musical Entertainment* occupies a high position in the therapeutic scale as the ease and extent of application combine qualities that are not of usual association. The instant appeal of a concert obviates any difficulties that may arise in otherwise securing the voluntary attendance of those patients who may be benefited as listeners; and the number of the latter, granted ample concert hall accommodation, will reach a very high percentage of the total hospital population, both male and female. In this manner, the disadvantage of limited application associated with the active type is more than counterbalanced by the simultaneous passive treatment of large numbers where the attention to details and organising effort associated with the latter are of negligible amount in contrast to the time and energy expended in the former.

An essential condition for a thorough and exhaustive development of both active and passive recreational treatment through musical entertainment is the organisation of a hospital orchestra or brass band, or preferably both, the former being more adapted for indoor performance and the latter better suited for outdoor purposes. There are very few hospitals that do not include among the patient population some qualified musicians, who can be induced to co-operate in the establishment of such a band or orchestra. The introduction of a few qualified members of the staff, apart from necessity, will tend to inspire in the patient members of the band, a very desirable self-confidence that has been either weakened or lost as a result of the pathological mental state present. These staff musicians will also prove useful in assisting or supervising some of the individual or group rehearsals and thus lighten the already heavy burden of the recreational therapist. The organisation of such an orchestra will solve the problem of providing suitable music for the patients' dances and other concerts, as well as for the annual athletic sports and other functions.

In summing up it cannot be overstressed that musical entertainment is a highly important therapeutic agent that should admit of maximum development in all its various forms and occupy a prominent position in any occupational therapy régime. Its reactions are expressed in an improved intellectual and emotional tone in the individual participants and in a a happier and more cheerful hospital atmosphere.

(6) *Cinema Shows*, to which are closely allied *Dramatic Performances*, rank almost of equal importance to musical entertainments as a form of diversional treatment. They may be regarded as a more skilled and professional type of dramatic peformance than amateur plays produced within the hospital, but are solely of the passive type. What has already been said of musical entertainment, applies equally to similar shows and the production of plays, where the characters are portrayed mostly by the patients. In the latter, the active type of treatment is exemplified, while the passive type embraces a wide range of application. Cinema shows, formerly of the silent type, are now almost exclusively of the spoken variety and the apparatus used for the latter can be converted for the reproduction of gramophone records, musical and otherwise, which enhance the value of such apparatus. Radio instruments, which are capable of reproducing wireless plays, as well as musical concerts, are similarly convertible for the transmission of gramophone concerts by means of a suitable 'pick-up' from records and if the radio programmes are transmitted to all parts of the hospital from a central machine by a network of speakers, gramophone concerts can, in this way, reach even a larger number of listeners than is possible in the concert hall. The installation of a talking-picture apparatus in the hospital concert hall should be a definite feature of every advanced recreational therapy department. The simplicity of organ-

ising regular programmes from the wealth of material that is now available, covering a wide field of music, drama, comedy, travel, educational and news pictures, amply justifies the financial outlay involved in the cost of apparatus and the provision of films. Cinema shows comprise the nearest possible approach to stage drama and comedy and, in addition, provide a very versatile range of entertainment.

There must be a definite and wise system of selecting suitable programmes, where the recommendations of the distributor companies will be subjected to a critical examination by the recreational therapist, based on either preview or sound and comprehensive newspaper review. The cinema market is annually flooded with numbers of pictures that have a definite deleterious effect on normal mental health and again many adjudged suitable for normals, or at the least non-harmful, may have no therapeutic value for disordered minds and, in fact, may cause reactions that tend to impede recovery. Sex films and weird, bizarre plots, as well as crude comedies, should be rejected, while news reels should be a feature of every programme, as they tend towards resocialisation and stimulate healthy interests.

(7) Bibliotherapy is simply treatment or curing through the medium of books or reading. It is of the active type when the individual does his own reading, through books, periodicals or newspapers and of the passive variety where group reading and *lectures* are availed of. The patient who reads his daily newspaper, while persistently opposing handicraft treatment, is as active a participant in occupational therapy as the patient who creates the most artistic piece of leatherwork or fancy stitchcraft. If, as sometimes happens, such a patient reads the news for a group of fellow-patients, he is, perhaps unconsciously, extending the therapeutic value of his daily occupation, not alone for himself, but for the passive members of his group.

This form of recreation necessitates the provision and equipment of a large library, containing at least 1,000 volumes, apart from a regular and constant supply of periodicals and newspapers. While the majority of the books should be of the fiction type, a small percentage should deal with biography, travel, history, science, etc. As with films, care must be taken in the selection of the volumes and clean, healthy literature only introduced, eliminating undesirable sex stories, weird fantastic plots and books that have a depressing effect. It will be necessary to train an occupational nurse to take complete charge of the library (in the absence of a qualified librarian) who, in turn, will be assisted by a number of patients to supervise and effect the proper distribution and return of the volumes. A special system of ward distribution must be devised to meet the needs of any particular hospital, as the co-operation of each ward charge nurse must be secured to ensure the efficient upkeep of the various books, while in a particular ward. Such a system becomes an inevitable necessity, as not all the patients, for physical or other reasons, can attend the reading room of the library and a lending arrangement of this kind will meet the difficulty. It does not seem necessary to stress the advantages to be attained through bibliotherapy. A suitable novel will often make all the difference in prolonged convalescence from a physical illness and sometimes will provide the only form of occupation in a refractory psychosis.

(8) *Social Entertainments*, among which may be included picnics, refer to the organisation of impromptu social evenings and gatherings, where a medley of games, music and vocal items are arranged in an impromptu manner, on somewhat similar lines to a soirée or social evening in a private house. Tables of bridge, whist, napoleon and other card games are interspersed with tables of chess, draughts, dominoes, ping-pong and similar table games. Orchestral or solo music is also added and occasionally these continuous items are interrupted by vocal solos, duets or quartets and solo dances and other items, such as recitations, group singing, dependent on the extent of talent available. In fact, the prior arrangement of one or two special attractions will not in any way reflect on the impromptu nature of the evening. A feature of such a gathering is that there is a complete air of informality permeating the whole atmosphere of the evening. Patients are free to join or take part in any game they have a particular penchant for or even sample as many games as they wish.

Members of the medical and nursing staff present should assist in furthering the informal and free-and-easy nature of the party by mingling with the various groups. They should take part in the different games and chat here and there with the patients, as well as contributing to the musical side of the programme, when talent permits. The proceedings usually terminate with light refreshments for all—an item which proves a very attractive feature and one which completes the socialising effect of such evenings.

A more elaborate and specialised type of such parties may be arranged for festive occasions, such as, Hallowe'en, 'Xmas period, New Year's Eve and special national feast days. The games and musical items should be followed by a short dance, with the vocal and other extras continued between the individual dances. Apart from the therapeutic aspect of such gatherings and their very resocialising influence, they help to fill the many voids, associated with hospital detention, as contrasted with home conditions. There is probably nothing that helps so much to break the monotony of hospital existence and provide the best possible substitute for the external amenities of normal life, than recreational treatment of this kind, and it should be a feature of the occupational therapy programme of every progressive and up-to-date hospital.

(9) *Walks and Hikes, Motor and Coach Drives, Sight-seeing Excursions*, etc., are other regular features of recreational programmes and add to the novelty and diversity of available entertainment. Walks and hikes should be almost daily features for small groups of suitable patients and can be availed of on most Sundays for further groups, who cannot be accommodated on week days. The routes chosen should be varied to avoid monotony, and where hikes are organised, a portable lunch should be arranged to increase the time necessary for such excursions. Not all patients will be found mentally or physically suited for these, especially for the latter, and fatigue should be avoided in all cases. Motor and coach drives should be organised monthly, if feasible, and trips arranged to the seaside where practicable, or to other accessible scenic beauty spots. One monster excursion

should be arranged each summer when the maximum possible number of patients should be given a complete day's outing.

(10) *Hobbies*, because of their diversional nature, are included in the recreational section, though many authorities regard them as a special unit of the handicraft division. The fact that they are of a diversional non-productive type of occupation, would appear to justify their separation from the more utilitarian and commercial section dealing with handicrafts proper. In other words, the money spent on the purchase of materials for any particular hobby is not recouped financially at any later stage beyond the vastly superior and incomparable therapeutic return achieved thereby, which latter cannot be measured in terms of financial units or permit of comparison with the monetary outlay involved.

In normal life the importance of acquiring a hobby outside one's daily avocation has been stressed from time immemorial. It is a sound substitute for what often transpires to be unhealthy introspection, which latter is often a very fertile breeding ground for many a psychoneurosis and even a psychosis. It avails of time that may be spent unproductively in worrying or brooding over difficulties—the forerunner of obsessional or depressive states. It fills up a void between the cessation of routine working hours and the time set aside for sleep, by the proper utilisation rather than the useless waste of one's spare time. The pursuit and cultivation of an interesting hobby is of definite mental-hygiene value in many other respects. It helps to engender a proper and broader perspective of life, inducing a physical and mental invigoration, so necessary for tackling the workaday problems of business. It prevents, as Winston Churchill has stated in his *Thoughts and Adventures*, wearing out part of one's mind by over-use, through the adoption of suitable rest, by acquiring other mental interests.

If all this be true for normals, how inestimable must the value of a hobby be in mental or physical illness, especially in cases of prolonged convalescence, where the monotony of enforced idleness must conduce to mental irritability and other undesirable psychical trends. Here, introspective and autistic activities are replaced by more healthy interests and the time given to day-dreaming and phantasy-formation is directed into more realistic and utilitarian channels. Life assumes a more interesting and hopeful form and a stepping-stone is provided across what must appear like a chasm between the world of disordered mentation and the real world outside.

There are myriads of hobbies to choose from for normals, but for environmental, economic and other reasons, these are naturally restricted for hospital use. In mental hospitals, the *Cultivation of Individual Garden Plots* can be permitted within limitations as to available space and choice allowed as to use. Some may concentrate on flowers, others on fruits and others still on vegetables, in accordance with individual taste. The range of cultivation should embrace indoor gardens, roof gardens, where possible, window boxes, rock gardens, etc. The *Caring of Various Animals*, such as birds, rabbits, poultry, etc., may prove an absorbing hobby as it does for many normals. *Philately* (stamp-collecting) is another intriguing hobby that has many devotees, and the work is not confined solely to collection. There is further occupation in sorting, arranging for page classification and then mounting, as well as exchanging stamps with fellow collectors. This interchange of part collections makes very desirable social contacts which add to the therapeutic side of this hobby. *Art-painting* can be a very attractive hobby for those with little previous ability and a worthy substitute, requiring less art in execution and yet reproducing with even more accuracy, is that of *Photography*. Here, given the necessary apparatus, a patient, with little tuition, can secure quite satisfactory results. *Modelling and Sculpture* may also come within the scope of a limited number of patients, even though the results lack professional finish. There may be many other hobbies of similar therapeutic value to supplement this list.

*Organisation and Personnel.* It has been the rule in many cases to place the recreational section under the control of a physical drill instructor, who may be an expert in physical training and who may or may not be conversant with the many other activities of this section. As there is much more involved in the treatment than mere physical culture and the principles underlying it being of a more comprehensive nature than that encompassed by the latter, it should be under the immediate direction of a *Recreational Therapist*, who will be responsible through the chief occupational therapist to the medical superintendent. The recreational therapist will have made a special study of the principles and practice of diversional treatment in all its details and will usually be an occupational therapist who has specialised in recreational treatment. Such an appointment is definitely recommended, as the duties attaching to the directorship of this section are of a wholetime nature and may also include the responsibility for the re-educational programme outlined in the next chapter.

The recreational therapist will find it useful to divide his department into (1) Outdoor Activities, (2) Indoor Activities and (3) Re-educational Section. It will be necessary to select the more apt and skilled members of the nursing staff, whom we will train as occupational nurses to take charge, under his direction, of each of these three divisions.

(1) *Outdoor Activities* embrace all forms of amusement held in the open air and are of a varied character, being classified into (a) *Extramural* and (b) *Intramural*, according as a particular recreation operates mainly outside the hospital estate, or within the hospital grounds.

(a) *Extramural Activities* would include walks, hikes, excursions, motor drives, picnics and any ball or other games played against outside teams at a non-home venue, as well as cinema and circus shows or concerts and such entertainments arranged specially at outside halls. Visits to local horse-race and greyhound-coursing meetings, dog-track races, football matches, athletic contests and other external sporting fixtures, providing purely passive amusement, would be similarly classified.

(b) *Intramural Activities* cover all forms of amusement organised in the open air within the hospital walls. This would include the annual athletic sports fixture, where contests in running, jumping, hurdling, weight-throwing, cycling, tug-o'-war, medley and novel events are arranged for both patients and staff. This athletic meet should be regarded as the annual hospital Gala Day and should be organised as elaborately as possible. The hospital brass band or substitute music from outside should occupy a prominent place in the programme and a large number of novel events, such as wheelbarrow races, egg and spoon races, sack races, obstacle races, etc., should be included to add to the humorous side of the day's sport. Suitable prizes should be secured for the winner and runner-up in each event and the presentation of the trophies should be arranged as a special ceremony at the conclusion of the meeting. In fact, no effort should be spared to make certain that the entire programme be modelled, as far as possible, on its prototype for normals. This duplication of external details tends to create environmental factors that help to reawaken dormant social interests of vast therapeutic importance. All members of the medical and nursing staffs, where possible, should attend this annual function.

Other intramural activities held in the open in the various exercise grounds of the hospital would embrace calisthenics, gymnastics, drills, field games of all types and open-air dances, when possible, as well as band promenades, etc. Arrangements should be made to hold the calisthenics and gymnastics programmes in the open as far as possible. Small group games and team games will also be arranged as circumstances permit, with interdivisional contests between different sections of the hospital. The development of team rivalry produces more interest and more serious attention will be devoted to the training practices in preparation for these contests. The acquisitive instinct to secure victory becomes the immediate objective, and carries with it the therapeutic purpose which is the real and all-important motive underlying the entire programme. Band promenades can also be arranged when weather permits. These can be made regular features of the recreational therapy department, which has been progressive enough to establish a brass band. Occasionally, the services of outside bands may be secured, whether one exists in the hospital or not.

(2) *Indoor Activities*, though not comparable to treatment in the open air, are the only means of dealing with the recreational problems, resulting from weather or seasonal restrictions. The increased confinement arising from a reduction of daylight hours in winter and the weather vagaries of all seasons can only be ameliorated by an alternative indoor programme arrangement providing for these factors. In any case, there are many commendable forms of amusement, both active and passive, that are of the indoor variety solely and some of these, such as cinema shows, have to be featured indoors, even when conditions are suitable for outdoor treatment. All indoor activities are divided into (a) *Central* and (b) *Ward*. The former refers to entertainments and functions held in the central recreational concert hall or the physical drill and calisthenics held in the latter in the absence of a special gymnasium. In addition to the two mentioned, central recreational activities include dances, social entertainments, concerts and musical shows, lectures, cinema shows, bridge and whist drives on large scale, dramatic performances, etc.

Dances should be a weekly feature during the winter months and should be arranged as a regular sequel to the usual items arranged for social parties on festive occasions already referred to. They should be of the mixed type, female and male patients being encouraged to dance with each other. Members of the nursing staff should not be permitted to partner each other, except for very special reasons. Folk dances and round dances should receive pride of place as they make more for socialisation and for reasons already enumerated.

Musical shows and concerts should be arranged as often as circumstances permit and there is no reason why suitable patient talent should not be introduced if available. Musical shows may be arranged by a central wireless broadcast, or by the screening of suitable musical films, or gramophone concerts may be provided by utilising the special record transmission apparatus attached to the sound film machine. To secure diversification and thus maintain interest, lectures, dramas and card drives should be staged. Lectures can be made attractive by choosing a suitable subject and a competent and humorous lecturer, who should arrange lantern slides for projection to illustrate the trend of the talk. The staging of plays and comedies, especially if purely hospital productions, will be received with far more enthusiasm than any other central function. The cast should be recruited, as far as possible, from patient talent with a limited number from the staff to balance the production and instil confidence. A few talented members of the staff, given key parts, will make for reassurance among the others, who may already be suffering from 'stage fright' in a psychological sense.

Card drives should be arranged at least monthly, on a large scale, and be of the mixed type as for normals. Bridge may not be within the competence of a sufficient number of patients to arrange a large drive, but whist which is easily learned, will be known to a large percentage of the patients. As many members of the staff as are available should be prevailed on to join in the drive and the usual quota of trophies, adapted to hospital needs, should be presented to the different score winners. Here again, as in all occupational therapy activities, the object aimed at should be the creation of an atmosphere of realism, so that interests and emotions that have become dormant should be reawakened by environmental influence.

Social entertainments, or as they are generally called, social evenings, should be at least a monthly function and held in the main central recreational hall of the hospital. Details of the different items arranged for the evening have already been enumerated and the general informal atmosphere that should prevail. There should be the largest possible attendance on the part of the medical and nursing staffs and all should take an active part in furthering the various amusements and thus contribute towards the evening's enjoyment. Such evenings should be organised on a more elaborate scale and followed by a dance on certain festive occasions as already suggested, introducing features, appropriate to the celebration of the particular festival, such as apple games on Hallowe'en and carol singing during the 'Xmas period, or on New Year's Eve.

Reference has already been made in detail to the advantages

of a central cinema talkie apparatus. This can be installed
in the main recreation hall, making the necessary alterations
to secure proper projection. Arrangments should be made
for the use of as large a screen as possible at the stage end
of the hall and the erection of a fireproof projecting box
at the other end outside the external wall. Owing to the
myriads of films and newsreels that are now available, there
should be little difficulty in arranging weekly programmes,
or at least fortnightly. One can also visualise a very forward
and progressive occupational therapy department acquiring,
or possibly constructing, the necessary apparatus—microphone, amplifier, revolving camera, etc., to record and reproduce with sound on the screen, local happenings, not
confined to hospital activities. There will be plenty of material
in the outdoor activities of the recreational department
whose sound and light reproductions will be a source of
added amusement, when such are included as a tit-bit in the
ordinary talkie programme. It has already been achieved in
silent film features and will probably be common-place
in talkie programmes of the future.

*Ward Activities* constitute the recreational facilities that
are provided in the different wards. Owing to weather conditions and the longer winter hours that have to be spent
indoor, arrangements must be made to secure a balanced
programme of handicraft and recreational therapy, both
for the patients who attend occupational centres outside
the ward and those who, for physical or mental reasons, are
restricted to ward treatment. Chief among ward amusements
are card, table and miniature indoor games of all types and
detailed reference has already been made to those. Calisthenics are also organised in the wards for similar reasons.
The deteriorated patients will engage in the first steps in
occupational treatment in the ward, through simple games
and calisthenics.

Probably in no section or unit of the treatment, of both the
handicraft and recreational type, will the complete co-
operation of the nursing staffs be so essential as in the development of the different ward activities. Here the entire success
of this section of the treatment will be dependent on the
goodwill and support of the ward nurses. They should all

enter into the proper spirit of the therapy and regard this form of treatment as one of primary concern. It is in the impromptu organisation of ward games that the nurse's resources and ability will be truly tested. It requires little prior instruction or skilled experience to induce the patient, who might otherwise be unoccupied, to take part in small group games or even those of an individual nature.

Musical entertainments can also be organised in the wards. It must be remembered that there is a large number of patients, apart from those confined to bed, who will not avail of the amusements organised in the recreation hall. For these, occasional ward concerts should be arranged as well as music recitals. A more or less permanent method of providing such musical and other entertainment is the provision of a large concert loud speaker in each ward, with a connection to a central radio apparatus, or, as an alternative, the provision of a small radio receiver in such wards, if the cost is not prohibitive. There can be no question that this very modern and novel form of supplying continuous entertainment has proved a wonderful boon and assistance in increasing recreational facilities in hospitals. A central receiving apparatus of the kind, has the additional advantage that gramophone recordings of all kinds can be amplified and transmitted through it, to all the wards' loud speaker instruments, by the use of a 'pick-up,' to replace the usual gramophone sound box. It is, in fact, possible to connect a suitable microphone to this radio apparatus and thus facilitate the broadcast to the wards of concerts, lectures and other entertainments held in the main recreational hall.

In a general textbook of occupational therapy, such as this, it is not possible to discuss, in more detail, the recreational activities of the O.T. department. The importance of this section of treatment is of such a nature as to justify the publication of a treatise dealing exclusively with it. The development of amusements, recreations, hobbies and diversions of all kinds, in a therapeutical system, involves activities of such a comprehensive nature, with such possibilities for extension to every section and part of a mental hospital, that a special textbook is essential to cover, adequately, every possible phase of this form of treatment.

# CHAPTER IX.

## SECTIONS AND UNITS (*contd.*)

### RE-EDUCATIONAL SECTION

RE-EDUCATION, in the occupational therapy sense, is the restoration of normal clean habits of living, in regressed psychotics, where these habits have been lost or replaced by bad ones, through a special system and method of training, akin to the process and course of normal education. Though normal education methods may be simulated, the training programme is definitely of the re-educational type and is merely super-imposed on a previous educational background, which has become disintegrated through the retrogressive influence of psychotic disease. This immediately excludes aments or mental defectives, whose education has not been along normal lines or reached normal standards. Re-education is, accordingly, a system of habit-training for deteriorated and regressed mental cases, who have developed habits of uncleanliness, untidiness and destructiveness. It tends to resuscitate decent social and bodily habits among this class of patients with the twofold purpose:

1. To initiate the rehabilitation of the deeply regressed patients with a view to restoring them to communal life, by means of the various grades of occupational therapy projects arranged, in a methodical manner, in the Habit-training Schedule.

2. To make them more acceptable and better-conducted members of the hospital community, where recovery or even remission, that would justify temporary communal sojourn, appears unattainable even after intensive and assiduous application of the treatment.

The vast majority requiring re-educational treatment of this kind is of the schizophrenic or dementia praecox variety, a mental disease, which, in itself, constitutes a large percentage of the psychotic conditions requiring mental hospital treatment. Schizophrenia, which Adolph Meyer referred to as a disease of disorganised habits, constitutes the main bulk of mental regression met with and is of four main varieties:— (1) Simple, (2) Hebephrenic, (3) Katatonic and (4) Paranoid. Modern teaching rightly views, with disfavour, the use of the term *Dementia* in these cases, replacing even the unsatisfactory term *Dementia Praecox* by the more generally approved title of *Schizophrenia* introduced by the German authority Bleuler in 1911. It is now agreed that the alleged *dementia* is not progressive in all cases to the extent stated. Some cases recover and many exhibit remission of symptoms for longer or shorter periods, while quite a large number reach an arrested state of regression of greater or lesser depth. Further, the association of adolescence and precociousness with the disease is not standard in all cases. It is well known that some cases develop long after the expiry of the adolescent period and the element of precocity is not constant in the histories of many of the cases. It was on this account that Bleuler rightly introduced the term *Schizophrenia*, which, derived from the Greek, means 'split mind.' It is this splitting of the psyche or mind that is advanced to explain the persistence of hallucinations in the disease. Kraepelin has advanced the following statistical returns: 75% of Hebephrenics reach profound dementia, while 17% become partially demented and are capable of much useful work under supervision and 8% make an apparent recovery.

60% of Katatonics reach advanced dementia; 27% reach an arrested stage and improve sufficiently to permit their being allowed home, while 13% show permanent or temporary recovery.

With regard to Dementia Paranoides, though short remissions may occur occasionally, temporary or permanent recovery is rare.

The Simplex type, which is really a persistence of a mild form of the disease, characterised mostly by mental apathy and lack of normal ambition, rarely progresses further beyond this stage and is not known to advance to any degree of extreme regression. It must, however, be borne in mind that these clinical subdivisions of the disease are based on the predominance of certain symptoms in each type—mental apathy in the simplex type, seclusiveness in hebephrenia, alternating phases of excitement, inertia and quiescence of symptoms with mannerisms, etc., in katatonia and hallucinations and delusions of persecution in the paranoid type. Patients, however, may pass from one type to the other or show features of two or more types of the disease simultaneously.

Contrary to the older acceptation, schizophrenic deterioration is of the emotional, rather than the intellectual type, and this is remarkably so in hebephrenia. There is no general intellectual impairment or mental enfeeblement of the type that one associates with the secondary or senile dementias. Otherwise, there would be no basis for the recoveries and remissions that are experienced in many cases, even after years of so-called *dementia*. It likewise accounts for the re-educational measures recommended for this type of regression and their inapplicability to other forms of mental deterioration.

The disease appears to be characterised by emotional disorder of both a positive and negative type. The former explains the apparent loss of the normal emotional function, which is an outstanding feature of the symptomatology of the condition, so well exemplified by the nonchalant and indifferent attitude displayed by such cases on receipt of news of the death of a very near relative. This failure of normal emotional response is merely an apparent loss of emotion. In such cases there is no true loss, merely a withdrawal of effect from conscious reality and its attachment to various unconscious repressed complexes. This splitting of consciousness is typical of the condition. Negative emotional disturbances account for the apparently senseless laughter and often alternate crying met with in many cases. There are, thus, two disorders of emotion encountered, *Athymia* or loss of normal emotional response and *Parathymia* or distortion or disharmony of emotion. The restoration of the normal emotional 'flow,' by creating constant contact with day to day realities, is the main concern of occupational therapy in general and re-educational therapy in particular.

As already defined, the immediate object of re-education is the resuscitation of normal habits of cleanliness and the substitution of more desirable habits for any unhygienic ones that may be acquired during the course of the psychosis. *Habit* is described as 'a new form of adjustment acquired during the lifetime of an individual' and thus excludes instinctive activity and congenital reflex reactions; a conditional reflex, on the other hand, is a definite example of habit-formation, and some authorities would explain all habit development through the establishment of such reflexes. Maher defines habit as an 'acquired aptitude for some particular mode of action' and explains that the facility for the performance of a particular act is increased by each repetition. This repetition and consequent facilitation forms the basis of all educational development and must be the guiding principle in any progressive form of re-educational therapy. It is responsible for developing the habits of walking, speaking, reading and writing and leads to skill and knowledge in the various crafts and professions. This theory of the *Association Psychologists* is based on the fact that the nervous system is provided with a series of innately organised motor mechanisms, consisting of motor neurones with axons leading to certain muscles and also provided with sensory nerve connections to one or more sense-organs, in such a way that stimulation of the sense-organ excites a nervous current, which passing through the motor mechanism, produces reflex movement, whether simple or complex, according to the number of muscles affected. If two or more of these motor mechanisms are thrown into action simultaneously or in immediate succession by the conjunction or succession of appropriate sense-stimuli, they become linked together by paths of low resistance in the nervous system and this linkage leads to the formation of habit. In this manner, a new motor mechanism is established by constant repetition, which eventually becomes what is described as 'secondarily automatic.' This is effected by combining our more elementary movements in many ways, by constant practice, developing habitual action or skilled movements. These secondarily automatic actions, described by the Scholastic Psychologists as 'habitually voluntary,' are thus distinguished from the 'primarily automatic' actions—the physiological reflexes, which are congenital. Gruender states that a 'neural organisation' is acquired by the mere repetition of an action. In proportion as this 'neural organisation' reaches perfection, the less voluntary attention to the external actions of the developing habit is exercised, until a stage is reached when the will to perform the details of the movements disappears, as occurs, for instance, when acquiring the skill or habit of cycling. When the latter becomes a purely habitual action, the mind can become engrossed in thoughts of an entirely different character, without having to concentrate on the movements associated with steering and pedalling. This explains the necessity for the sense of sight in the early stages, when acquiring the skill of cycling, as most beginners fail to cycle in the dark in the early developing stage of the habit. Scholastic Psychologists have defined habit ('habitually voluntary' action) as one that is due to a past action of the will (*imperium voluntatis*) to which, however, we no longer pay any attention. They must distinguish it from an 'actually voluntary' act and recognised between the two as end stages many transitional stages which they designated as the 'gradual mechanisation of voluntary actions.' This is a very apt and intelligible description of the method of procedure in habit-formation and offers a very sensible rationale in the development of re-educational treatment.

James, Woodworth and Spencer, all famous psychologists, regarded habits as acquired instincts, which only differ from innate or congenital instincts in their genesis or origin. James, in addition, held that instincts were merely transitory, forming the basis or groundwork of habit, by which they ultimately became supplanted. McDougall states that acceptance of this theory would endow habits with the impulsive powers of instincts and is of opinion that habit has no motive power—'the habitual action,' he says, 'is only purposive when performed in the service of a purpose with the origin of which it has nothing to do.'

Habits have been generally classified on a physiological basis into:—

1. Habits of mind, such as punctuality, etc.

2. Habits of body, where the body adapts itself to climatic or other changes, such as exercise or variations in diet, etc.

3. Habits of intellect, such as the habitual use of certain words or phrases in daily conversation.

Based on the presence or absence of sensory discrimination of stimuli in the performance of habitual actions, habits are divided broadly into (a) *Motor* and (b) *Sensory*. In the former, emphasis is placed on the motor reaction, while in the latter it is placed on the stimulus which causes the reaction, otherwise there is no essential difference between the two. *A Motor Habit* is therefore an acquired method of reaction of a special type in response to a specific stimulus. Thus, most people have acquired the habit of loosening a nut on a bolt by turning it anti-clockwise and the chief element of the entire action is purely motor, but when sensory discrimination is brought into play, as occurs when removing the nuts or studs attaching wheels to left-hand threaded hubs, the action is reversed and one has to discriminate as to the use of correct stimuli. This latter would be described as a sensory habit, as the element of sensory discrimination becomes the emphasised feature additional to the motor activities, which are common to both. *A Sensory Habit* would, accordingly, be described as an acquired method of reaction in response to one particular stimulus, rather than another or others of the same general type. A third type of habit, called the *Delayed Reaction* type, is also described, but this is merely a motor or sensory habit, where the customary reaction takes place only after a short interval of from part of a second to possibly some days after the stimulus excitation. This is exemplified in the daily routine of replying to correspondence at some interval after receipt—perhaps some hours later or the next day. It is noteworthy that the vast majority of habitual actions are of the delayed type, though such habits are not acquired as promptly as those where the reaction succeeds the stimulus almost instantaneously. This latter is one of the first of the more important rules in habit-formation which must receive due recognition in any properly planned scheme of re-education.

### Rules in Habit Formation

There are certain principles or rules in the development of habits which must be recognised to ensure success in re-educational measures. The first, just referred to, states that the occurrence of an interval between the specific stimulus and the appropriate reaction, will affect the speed with which a habit may be acquired. The greater the interval, the longer it will take to form the habit; hence instantaneous reaction methods are paramount in habit-training.

*Secondly*, habit-formation is also governed by the frequency and number of the learning periods. Psychological experiments with animals have demonstrated that it requires a certain number of days with one trial each day to train an animal to develop a particular skill, while another animal allowed two trials each day will acquire the same habit in somewhat more than half the time. In the second case, the number of trials are actually increased and the rest intervals are reduced. It is evident, therefore, that short training sessions, with definite free intervals, increase the rapidity of habit acquirement.

*Thirdly*, the greater the number of movements to be taught and the finer the adjustments that have to be made, the more difficult it becomes to implant the habit. Conversely, the fewer and more gross the movements, the quicker the habit is acquired.

*Fourthly*, the idiosyncrasies of the patient and the profundity of mental regression present, as well as the chronicity of the condition under treatment, will influence the success or otherwise of the re-educational measures adopted. The latter point, as to the chronicity of the psychosis, will be dealt with further on in the conditions laid down for the selection of the patient material for the training classes. Some patients will respond to treatment much more rapidly than others, as the training procedures will prove more difficult for the less receptive members of the class.

*Fifthly*, and lastly, the entire daily re-educational programme must be a balanced régime of work, play and rest, covering a 24 hour schedule, with provision for graduation not unlike the educational system of class promotion in primary schools.

These subsidiary principles of occupational therapy are in the nature of rules of guidance in the development of the re-educational section and must be observed to ensure maximum results. They are supplemented by a number of conditions that might also be regarded as subsidiary principles in dealing with patients for the various training classes and the arrangements for their progress during treatment. These conditions are tabulated as follows:—

(1) Only patients classed as *Grade* 1 are suitable for the habit-training classes and will be promoted to *Grade* 2 if they have sufficiently benefited by the treatment after the required period. This presupposes the division of all suitable mental cases into three broad groups, based on the severity of mental symptoms and the intellectual capacity present in relation to occupational therapy in general, with a view to providing a stepping-stone arrangement in the treatment.

*Grade* 1 would include all the regressed schizophrenics and such deteriorated types, who require more or less individual attention, owing to the development of destructive and bad habits, with general evidence of lowered mentality. They are, at most, only suitable for very elementary craft and recreational treatment and provide the selective material for recruitment to the re-educational or habit-training classes. They are the type submitted for the first step or kindergarten section of a properly graduated occupational therapy department. The use of the word 'kindergarten' here does not imply dealing with children, but refers to the methods of infant training for application to adults, whose regressed mentalities resemble, in many respects, those of children. These regressed types have assumed a childlike attitude towards life, necessitating some substitute for parental guidance and supervision, and are very definitely capable of being taught anew, commencing with a kindergarten programme, not at all unlike that in use for children. The bad and destructive habits, normally associated with the infantile period, which are a feature of cases classed as *Grade* 1, must be subjected to the same kindergarten system of eradication and replacement.

*Grade* 2 consists of all those patients who have progressed from the re-educational section and all those whose mental comprehension is beyond the kindergarten or simple range of occupations and recreations. It would comprise those, who, though confined normally to the wards for one reason or another, are capable of doing more advanced work and taking part in simple card games and the less intricate games of skill, such as ring and deck quoits, table skittles, etc. They would perform most of the duties attaching to ward work and the manufacture of rugs or mats in wool, coir, etc. Tasks in simple basketry would come within their competence. They would constitute the material for the second step in occupational treatment.

*Grade* 3 would include all those who have graduated from Group 2, or the second step of the treatment, who are capable of engaging in the advanced crafts and recreations. They would comprise the convalescent types awaiting discharge home and those chronic cases, where recovery does not seem possible, but who have been trained to undertake skilled work, either at the special occupational therapy centre, the trades shops or other utility sections, such as the laundry, farm, etc. All these patients would have progressed from the Ward O.T. or special Ward O.T. centres to reach this, the third or final step in the treatment.

(2) The chronicity of the disease must be taken into account in the selection of cases, as well as the age in each individual case. Patients who exceed 40 years of age should not be selected for habit-training, as, apart from the diminished receptivity encountered in such cases, the retarded execution of movement and activity in general would obstruct the smooth running of the daily schedule for the younger and more agile members of the class, and the progress of the class generally would be impeded by the extra individual attention that would have to be expended in such cases.

Likewise, a psychosis of long standing would be a definite

contraindication for re-educational treatment and it is generally agreed that only cases of 10 years' duration or less should be permitted to join any habit-training class. The longer the psychosis, the more fixed the deteriorated habits have become and consequently the greater the difficulty in eradication. Further, the younger the patient, the easier it is to inculcate new habits of life.

(3) Patients suffering from any form of chronic physical disease should not be included in a habit-training class and even ill-health of a temporary nature should receive prior attention. This, accordingly, excludes any patient acutely ill, as the daily programme is of the active type and all members of the class must be physically fit to avoid individual lagging, which would lead to a general retardment in the class progress anticipated. This does not exclude patients naturally mute or suffering from mutism, if they understand the orders given and execute them with average efficiency.

(4) Habit-training classes should not consist of more than ten patients—the smaller the number, the greater the amount of individual attention exercisable. Small classes in addition to providing more individual attention, permit of more intensive application of the treatment and decrease the tendency towards distraction among the members of the class. A minimum of six, however, is advisable, as the repetition of movements in many of the exercises brings the imitative instinct into play, where verbal orders and passive movements might not possess the same influence.

(5) The segregation of the classes in a special isolated section of the hospital is a very necessary condition. A self-contained building, with exclusive, even if limited, outdoor recreational facilities, is the optimum arrangement for a re-educational class, where possible. In the absence of such a special cottage or unit, segregation should permit of a special dayroom, diningroom and dormitory, with a suitable exercise ground as adjacent as possible. Both dayroom and recreation ground must be suitably equipped to provide for all phases of the re-educational programme.

(6) Finally, all patients must be submitted for treatment

only on medical prescription. The appropriate prescription card must be completed in each case by the medical officer placed in charge of this section of the O.T. department, who selects the cases for each class and subsequently reviews those who, after a period of at least three months' treatment, do not appear to have progressed. These latter can be transferred to another class just commencing treatment, or the medical officer may advise against further re-educational treatment in some cases.

### Personnel:

The section should be in charge of a re-educational therapist, who is a fully qualified occupational therapist, versed in the principles and practice of re-educational treatment. The personnel of the nursing staff assisting in the treatment will require careful selection and subsequent tuition to appreciate the main principles and working details. The success or otherwise of the section will depend largely on their sympathetic co-operation. This is especially true of the nurse in charge of the unit, whose promotion to that of occupational (re-educational) nurse will follow from the results achieved, but all nurses attached to the unit must mutually assist in carrying out the daily schedule. In fact, as the entire daily programme covers 24 hours, the less active details of the treatment in the late evening, early morning and during the night will be solely in the hands of the nursing staff, both day and night. Much will, therefore, depend on the conscientious manner in which they will operate their respective details of the schedule, as they will be in sole charge during the periods mentioned. If they do not develop a sympathetic understanding of the principles and end-results of the treatment, even after due and careful selection for the work, they should be replaced. Any alteration in time, or details, of the programme arranged by the therapist, would otherwise have an adverse effect on the good results achieved during other periods of the daily schedule. It will, therefore, be appreciated how necessary it is to exercise great pains and care in the selection of the necessary staff, noting that patience and enthusiasm are the outstanding qualities required to undertake supervision of habit-training classes.

## The Daily Re-educational Schedule

As this schedule is of the continuous type, covering the daily 24 hours, it is obviously impossible to lay down a standard programme to be observed in every mental hospital. Variations in the number of sleeping hours and the hours for meals in the different hospitals will operate against the adoption of a standardised schedule. It is proposed here to arrange a schedule that will be concerned chiefly with the recognition of the principles and general balance of the programme, and it should be possible for each hospital to adapt it so as to conform with local time-table requirements without altering the general features:—

8 *a.m.* Each patient rises out of bed and immediately turns the upper bed-clothes completely over end-rail at foot of bed. Commences to dress, putting on trousers, socks and slippers, leaving pyjamas or night-shirt, as the case may be, unfolded on bed.

Immediately following three rings on special gong, members of the class proceed to lavatory for personal toilet—this consists of urination, followed by putting on and closing of shoes, replacing slippers in locker, washing face and hands and subsequently teeth, and returning to dormitory to complete dressing, including combing and brushing of hair, etc. The carrying out of these and all other details of the treatment is supervised by the nurse or nurses in charge under the guidance of the re-educational therapist. Actual physical assistance in promoting essential passive movements may be necessary, particularly in the early stages in each class. With dress and toilet complete, all patients line up for dress parade and corrections made when necessary and are then taken for a short but not brisk walk of not more than 15 minutes' duration—this is replaced by gentle calisthenics when weather is unfavourable, finishing with march, in single or double file, to refectory or diningroom for breakfast.

9 *a.m.* Breakfast. This must be consumed slowly, due

reference being paid to the inculcation of proper table manners —all bolting and messing of the food being prevented. Grace before and after meals must be said aloud, if possible by one of the patients. Immediately after breakfast, all return to ward in single or double file as permissible, and relax in a state of complete rest till 10 a.m. This arrangement for relaxation after meals, of shorter duration in the case of the minor meals, and of at least one hour in the case of the chief meal, while an important principle in the matter of dietetic hygiene for normals must be an essential part of any re-educational scheme, as providing the requisite balance between work, play and rest.

*Following gong at* 10 *a.m.* All attend lavatory for personal toilet and subsequently wash hands. Return to dormitory, make beds, tidying up in ward and dormitory with general ward work, brushing, dusting, polishing, etc. All patients, in addition to being taught habits of personal cleanliness and tidiness at all times, must be enjoined to keep their living quarters orderly and neat. The development or rather the resuscitation of these habits form an important socialising link in the general therapeutical chain of re-education.

10.30 *a.m.* Twice weekly, but at least once each week, all patients are to have fully immersed warm baths on fixed day or days, to be followed by shaving, if required. Patients must be trained to make all the necessary preparations, undressing and subsequently dressing, brushing hair, and cleaning teeth, etc. On non-bathing days, if daily bath is not possible, this period is allotted to simple calisthenics, drills and marches, outdoors, if possible, progressing weekly to more advanced movements and skills, when general progress justifies it, till approximately 12.30 p.m.

12.40 *p.m.* Following short rest for 10 or 15 minutes, on sound of gong at 12.40 p.m., all attend at lavatory for personal toilet, followed by washing of hands and face, brushing of hair and general attention to appearance for subsequent dress parade before marching to the refectory for dinner as for breakfast.

1 *p.m.* Dinner in special diningroom arranged for all meals, to be served and eaten as directed for breakfast.

1.30 *p.m.* Return in single or double file to dayroom and complete relaxation and rest till at least 2.30 p.m.

*Following gong at* 2.30 *p.m.* All attend at lavatory for personal toilet, urination, washing of hands, etc., in preparation for handicraft treatment.

2.45 *p.m.* Handicraft Therapy. This is graded from the most elementary tasks in the early stages, such as simple papercraft, cutting and folding, sand-papering wooden articles, rag teasing, simple stitchcraft and gradually introducing more skilled work according to progress made, such as rug making, raffiacraft and basketry, needlecraft and subsequently rake knitting, and simple weaving, when further progress would mean promotion to Grade 2 for more advanced work. Most of the crafts mentioned here are for internal operation, but these can be substituted occasionally by such work in the open as sawing and cutting logs, carting with hand and wheel-barrows, pushing roller on lawns and avenues, simple gardening, etc.

*Following gong at* 4 *p.m.* Before tea, all patients attend at lavatory for urination and general toilet, including washing of hands and face, etc. Tea and light refreshments are then served to each patient as a reward for co-operation in the treatment. All relax and rest till 4.30 p.m., when recreational therapy is applied.

4.30 *p.m.* Recreational Therapy. This is conducted outdoors, whenever possible, and consists of elementary games, competitive and otherwise, including the medicine ball and simple games, as well as other suitable forms of the treatment. Variation is important to heighten and maintain interest. This concludes at, approximately, 5.45 p.m. Following gong, all attend at lavatory for urination and general toilet in preparation for dress inspection at 5.55 p.m. and march to dining-hall for supper at 6 p.m.

6 *p.m.* Supper in dining-hall with the same propriety and attention to detail and manners as at all other meals, returning in double or single file to ward at 6.30 p.m. and rest till 7 p.m. when other recreational activities are indulged in, of the passive type generally, concert, talkie and wireless programmes, etc., till 8.15 p.m.

*Following gong at* 8.15 *p.m.* All return to lavatory for toilet, urination, etc., and subsequently prepare for bed, undressing, etc. Lights out at 9 p.m.

At 11.30 p.m., 2 a.m., 4.30 a.m. and 6.30 a.m., all bed-wetters, generally segregated together, are taken to lavatory for urination by the members of the night nursing staff responsible. The number of these toilet periods at night is increased or decreased, on medical direction, according to the progress reported in each individual case.

It will be noted that practically every minute of the daily schedule is arranged methodically to externalise the patient's attention from self to his surroundings as the only practical antidote to self-centring and introspection so much a feature of the regressed psychotic. His entire day is made active and busy by a balanced arrangement of work, rest and play and he is induced back to a more normal type of life under the influence of direction, imitation and instinct, just as the infant is dealt with and with the same exactions of time, perseverance and patience.

As already pointed out, this form of treatment, during the greater part of the scheduled period, will be exclusively under the control of individual nurses. Its success will depend, therefore, on a rigid adherence to the operation of every single item outlined in the schedule, both in regard to time and individual detail. This will be so, particularly, in the late evening and during the night and early morning and those responsible for the treatment during these periods will require to give the fullest co-operation and assistance, so as to prevent any interruption in the continuity of the schedule.

# CHAPTER X.

## SECTIONS AND UNITS *(contd.)*

### COMMERCIAL SECTION

THE BASIC PRINCIPLE, underlying the application of all forms of occupational treatment, stresses the therapeutic side as primary and all other considerations as secondary thereto. This has been elaborated already in detail and constantly referred to throughout the text, almost to the extent of being considered a *repetitio ad nauseam.* The *sine qua non* importance of this guiding principle justifies the risk of such a critical appellation, apart from the necessity of further reference here, when introducing discussion of the commercial or business side of the treatment. The importance of the economic factor must not, however, be disregarded and should occupy a prominent, even if secondary position in any treatise on occupational therapy. Many enthusiasts consider a discussion of commercial methods as entirely out of place and contrary to the spirit of the treatment. For them there exists no necessity to correlate occupational therapy and sound business methods. The scientific side must not, they argue, be impeded by financial considerations. Anyone with a definite practical experience in the development and organisation of occupational therapy will appreciate the fallaciousness of such reasoning. These two aspects, theoretically so divergent and opposed, are in actual practice in close alliance and any fully developed occupational therapy department will demonstrate the close linkage between the two. Where ample provision is made for a successful and exhaustive application of the treatment with its various hospital ramifications, investigation will reveal that the treatment is operated on the most modern and up-to-date commercial system. This blending of the two is depicted by the black and red lines in the diagram, giving the personnel and sections of the treatment in chapter 5.

The commercial side of occupational therapy may be suitably discussed under three broad heads, (1) *Purchases*, (2) *Sales* and (3) *Records*, including Book-keeping, Secretarial and Clerical work, as well as Report Books and Prescription Cards.

### 1. *Purchases*

The organisation of all sections of the treatment, Handicraft, Recreational, etc., will involve the purchase of many and varied articles of equipment, particularly in the early stages and the continued purchase of materials to operate the different items of equipment, when installed. Purchases may, therefore, be considered under the two sub-heads of (a) *Equipment* and (b) *Materials*.

There are many crafts and occupations requiring special equipment and machines, but the following list embraces the vast majority of those generally constituting the handicraft activities of a well-developed O.T. department. The purchase of all these items of equipment listed involves a huge outlay running into four-figure costs and should be spread over a number of years, introducing some of the more essential crafts at first and gradually adding to these each year, according as the different sections become organised and expand to full development.

(a) *Equipment* consists of the various items of machinery essential for the operation of the different crafts, as well as articles required for Recreational and Re-educational purposes. A general summary of the more usual items of equipment would be classified under (1) *Handicraft*, (2) *Recreational* and (3) *Re-educational*. (1) In the development of crafts, the following items are standard in most O.T. departments:—*Looms* (Tweed, Carpet, Blanket, Coir, Table, etc.) for weaving craft, as well as many associated accessories, such as warping frames, beaming machines, raddles, heddles, shuttles, etc. *Knitting Machines* of different kinds (round for socks and flat for garments, etc.) and essential accessories, including overlock machines, skein winders, bobbin winders, ironing machines, etc. *Matting Frames* for the manufacture of coir and other mats in the following types: pile, skeleton, reversible, etc. *Wirecraft Machines* for manufacture of wire fencing, wire springs and hooks, etc. *Papercraft Machinery*, including book-binding equipment as follows: Printing Machines (Platen and Presses) with all the necessary accessories, type, chases, galleys, furniture, ink, planers, quoins, tweezers, line cutters, gouges, chisels, rubbing pads, ink rollers, composing sticks, guillotines, cutters, stitching machines, perforators, bodkins, awls, eyeletting pliers, hand punchers, scissors, saws, bone-folders, set squares, finishing stoves, pastes, stitching frames, book-binding presses and boards, gumming machines, finishing presses, planes, stencil brushes and cutters, etc. *Cardboard Machinery*, mitre cutters, slotters, punching machines, treadle cutters, scoring and bending machines, hand and treadle press machines with steel blanking cutters (these latter are also used in the manufacture of rubber mats and envelopes, etc). *Woodworking Machines*, such as band saws, planers, sanders, saw benches, drilling and mortising machines, turning lathes, carpenter's tools, etc. *Cementcraft Machinery*, consisting of slab and block machines, roof and floor tile machines, sewer pipe moulds, fence post and other special moulds, hand concrete mixers, etc. *Brushcraft Equipment* for set and drawn work, including pitch melters, special wood-boring machines, cutters, etc. *Basketry Implements*, such as knives, bodkins, rapping irons, bradawls, screwblocks, pliers, drills, hammers, clippers, shears. *Dyecraft Equipment*, including dye-tanks, mixers, janting tools for batch dyeing, pricking wheel for tracing, drying frames, etc. *Leathercraft Tools*, such as modellers, tracers, knives, spacers, eyelet-fixers, press stud tools, punch pliers, punches, hammers, etc. *Pokercraft Equipment*, including electric and other type poker machines. *Pottery Tools*, such as electric, gas or other kinds, potter's wheels (electric and foot), spray glazing apparatus, scrapers, cutters, sponges, bins, brushes, sieves, etc. *Pewter and Metal-work Tools*, hammers, stake heads, pliers, various saws, mallets, etc.

It is advisable to commence with those crafts and occupations that meet the economic requirements of the hospital, such as basketry, brushcraft, woodcraft, mat and carpet-making, as well as weaving, cementcraft, etc., where the resultant products replace former purchases from outside sources. These crafts can be supplemented by minor ones, such as leathercraft, knitting and stitchcraft, where cost of equipment is of negligible proportions.

In all cases the capital cost may be considerably reduced by soliciting an extensive range of quotations from all firms interested. Valuable information with regard to addresses of manufacturers, etc., may be secured from appropriate Trade Journals and Directories. Some journals, in fact, will supply, on written request, an exhaustive list of manufacturers dealing with any particular type of machine or article. Enquiries should, in addition, extend to overseas and Continental makers, if only for comparative price purposes. In any case, one cannot over-emphasise the absolute importance of adopting, in all cases, a system of exhaustive enquiry before finally deciding on the purchase of any item of equipment. In the matter of purchasing equipment, one must keep in mind the possibility of manufacture in the pre-existing technical sections of the hospital, such as the engineering and wood-working shops. Likewise, the possibility of purchasing secondhand equipment must not be lost sight of. This is especially true of wooden hand-looms of all kinds and many weaving and spinning accessories, as well as several reconditioned machines and steel products.

Consideration must also be given to the quality of the articles purchased. It is false economy to purchase a cheaper or cheapest quality in any article. Due heed must be paid, therefore, to the quality of the purchase, as well as the reputation of the proposed manufacturer. A good quality machine, even though reconditioned, when purchased from a reputable firm, with guarantees, is often a better proposition than a new article when offered by a firm of lesser-known repute.

Many items of equipment are on offer in different sizes, notably looms, and here one must be guided by the work to be done and the section where the machine is to be installed. In the case quoted, if the loom is required for ward-occupation purposes, a table loom or other small simple timber-made handloom is indicated. If on the other hand it is to be used in the Special Occupational Therapy Weaving Centre, then a more intricate steel, hand or pedal loom may be necessary and the type will be dependent on the articles to be produced, whether it be blankets, tweeds, cocoa-matting, etc.

(b) *Materials:* What has already been stressed in the purchase of equipment, applies, with equal force, to the provision of materials for the continuous operation of the equipment. Due consideration must be given to the quality of the raw materials required, as well as the integrity and reputation of the supplier, who should, if possible, be the immediate manufacturer. In all cases, samples should be invited, with quotations, to permit of comparative tests, in both quality and costings, and this latter is greatly facilitated by requesting, in all quotations, inclusion of freight charges to local rail centre. Many firms are wont to quote delivery charges forward to purchaser, unless otherwise requested, and much valuable time may be lost in computing the comparative costs of such quotations.

Quantitative, as well as qualitative, considerations also enter into the question of the purchase of raw materials. It is generally well known, in the commercial world, that the percentage discount allowed in sales transactions is proportionate to the extent of the order. In other words, it is more economical to buy in ton, rather than pound quantities, and one can secure ten tons of material at a cheaper rate than one ton. In this respect, however, one must be guided by the amount of store space available, as well as the bulkiness, or otherwise, of the material required. The routine policy should aim at maximum quantities in individual orders, consonant with sufficient storage and the perishability or otherwise of the materials. The difference in price involved may quite often be the only insurance against the loss entailed in the faulty handling of some of the materials by many psychotics, inexperienced as they generally are, particularly in the early stages, in bringing the finished products up to saleable standards.

As emphasised, this system of purchasing may involve

problems in storage beyond the normal capacity of a hospital,
even after utilising the extra storage space provided in the
basement of the Special Occupational Therapy Building.
The ultimate saving in cost, per annum, however, will
justify a close detailed examination of the problem, even
to the extent of providing new storage buildings, and the
cost of these latter may be completely liquidated by the
substantial savings achieved in individual orders. This
saving will range from ten per cent to as much as fifty per
cent in some items and constitute all the difference between
wholesale and retail buying. In such construction work,
many sections of the O.T. department may contribute, to
no small degree, in meeting what might otherwise be regarded
as a prohibitive building cost. This will be particularly
true of the cementcraft section, which will provide, at much
less than wholesale cost, such essential building materials
as concrete blocks, concrete floor and roof tiles, etc. The
woodworking section will similarly provide doors, windows,
presses, shelving, etc. This additional storage space will
also be necessary to house the finished products, prior to
sale and despatch, whether to the hospital or to outside
purchasers.

A comprehensive list of the type of materials in general
demand by O.T. departments would include the following
raw and semi-raw materials: *Wool*, teased and unteased;
*Woollen Yarns*, dyed and undyed, such as knitting, weaving,
carpet yarns, etc; *Coir Fibre* and *Coir Yarns* in various
strengths according to requirements; *Cotton*, *Linen* and
*Silk Yarns*; *Galvanised Wire* in various gauges ranging from
8 to 16 and in various qualities, dependent on purposes
required, whether for the manufacture of wire fencing, wire
mattresses, springs, lampshade-frames, etc. *Paper* in all
qualities and colours, including *Manilla*, light for the manufacture of envelopes, heavy for index card guides, folders,
etc. *Tinted Paper* for printing of all types, *Brown Kraft*
and *Common Brown* for wrapping and manufacture of paper
bags, etc; *Cardboard*, both straw and manilla, plain and
coloured for the manufacture of cardboard boxes, book-
binding, etc; *Timber* of all kinds, red and white deal, oak,

mahogany, walnut, lime, birch, beech, ash, teak, pine, plywoods, etc.; *Cementcraft Materials*, Portland Cement for making cement blocks, concrete fence posts, concrete sewer pipes, etc.; coloured cements for making floor and roof tiles, etc.; *Brushcraft Materials*, African and Bahia Bass, Grey Union and Coir Fibre for making floor brushes, Bassein for scrubbing brushes, Mexican Whisk for carpet brushes, and bristles for tooth brushes. All those fibres may be supplied out in lengths to requirements. Other brush-making materials include pitch for set work and wire for drawn work with suitable stocks bored and finished from the woodworking section, as well as handles; *Basketcraft Materials*, willows in varying strengths, cane from $1\frac{3}{4}$ mm. to $3\frac{3}{4}$ mm. sizes for weaving, $4\frac{1}{2}$ mm. to 8 mm. for staking, bases, handles, etc., and 12 mm. to 18 mm. for frames. While the purchase of cane in all sizes is unavoidable for most hospitals, suitable willows can be provided from the hospital farm, following cultivation of the proper type of willow plants in suitable ground, that is generally not required for agricultural purposes. *Dyecraft Materials*, consisting mainly of basic coal tar dyes, as well as some vegetable dyes and associated mordaunting and other auxiliary materials, such as gall powder, gum arabic, acetic and sulphuric acids, etc.; *Leathercraft Materials*, leather of all kinds, hides, fancy and gloving leathers, including morocco, calf skins, skivers, thonging, all in plain and colours, as well as accessory dyes and stains, press studs, zipp fasteners in various lengths and colours, etc.; *Pottery Materials*, chiefly clays and glazes. *Metalwork* and *Pewtercraft Materials*, including sheet pewter and pewter solder, burnishing powder, sheet brass, tin, copper, silver and steel with appropriate soldering materials, wire, rivets and suitable patina, etc.

To the foregoing list, covering the more usual crafts, must be added a host of other materials, auxiliary to these crafts, including *Rubber*, coloured and plain, for the manufacture of mats, some of the latter may be reclaimed from discarded rubber motor tyres, etc.; *Felts* and *Cloths* for bookbinding and *soft toy manufacture*, including accessories, such as artificial eyes, buttons, hair, special fittings, etc.; *Chinese* or *Sea Grass*, as well as rushes for covering stools and chairs manufactured in the woodworking section, as well as *Paints, Stains* and *Polishes* for finishing all woodwork products, including wooden toys, etc.; *Twines* and *Cording* for upholstery and nettingcraft, including macrame, jute and manilla; *Raffia*, natural and coloured for general raffia work; *Beads* and *Cork Mats* for beadcraft, etc.; *Cotton Canvas Netting*, for rug manufacture and raffia work; *Gesso Powder* and *Paints*, as well as *Gesso Paste* for Gesso Craft. Special *Linen, Woollen, Cotton* and *Jute Yarns* are also required for the special sections of weaving craft and knitting craft such as embroidery, crochet work, lacecraft, etc. In addition, *Mild Steel Bars* in varying strengths may be required for manufacturing special reinforcing material in concrete construction of all kinds and *Special Steel Fittings*, whether standard or made to special specification, may be necessary for the completion of many wood-working products. A brief list of these would include such items as folding card table fittings, hinges of all types, locks, accessory steel fittings for toy manufacture, such as pedal motor chassis and wheels, steel axles, brass and steel screws and plates and furniture fittings of all kinds. An important activity in the dyecraft section—the manufacture of inks of all types—will necessitate the purchase of such essential materials as *Bottles* and *Jars*, as well as suitable *Corks* and *Screw Caps*, whether made in wood, metal or bakelite.

(2) *Equipment and Materials for the Recreational Therapy Section* also require special consideration. The purchase of apparatus, essential for many games and sports, while not approaching the much more elaborate requirements of the Handicraft Section, will be as extensive as the range of therapeutic recreations to be availed of. The following may be cited as among the chief recreations for which equipment, whether simple or complex as the case may be, must be provided:—

(a) *Dancing, Musical Entertainments, Cinema Shows, Dramatic Performances, Concerts*, etc., will all necessitate the erection of a large recreational hall, fully equipped with stage, stage fittings, dressing-rooms, ballroom floor, etc., while equipment and materials appropriate to each, such as *Musical Instruments, Cinema Projection Apparatus, Costume,* and *Dresses*, etc., for drama production, *Ballroom Powders*, etc., must be purchased as required.

(b) *Gymnastics* demand various items of equipment, such as *Horizontal* and *Parallel Bars, Dumb-Bells, Bar-Bells, Indian Clubs, Vaulting-Horse*, etc.

(c) *Outdoor Games* and *Athletics* involve a medley of special apparatus and equipment, among which may be listed: *Special Attire, Hurdle* and *Jump Standards*, as well as many other items of general athletic equipment, balls and the various additional equipment associated with the different ball games, among which may be cited—Sticks and Bats for field games, such as Baseball, Golf, Hurling, Handball, Hockey, Cricket, Shinty, Lacrosse, Tennis, etc. In addition, quite a large number of field games necessitate special equipment appropriate to each, such as goalposts and other scoring posts, as well as flags, wickets, special nets, marking-machines, suitable play-pitches and courts for each game, etc.

(d) *Indoor Games* will call for a wide medley of apparatus and equipment, chief among which may be listed—playing-cards of all types, card-tables as well as equipment for billiards, table-tennis, chess, draughts, dominoes, quoits, skittles, etc., etc.

(e) *Bibliotherapy* will necessitate the development of a library and reading rooms, equipped with a wide range of suitable books, magazines and reading material of all kinds. This section of recreational treatment will have to budget annually for an adequate financial sum to provide for the purchase of suitable weekly and monthly magazines, particularly the illustrated types, daily and weekly newspapers, as well as new books and replacement of discarded or worn-out editions.

(f) *Hobbies*, such as photography, philately (stamp-collecting), individual garden-plot cultivation, etc., will each necessitate the purchase of appropriate equipment and materials. The latter, as with handicraft materials, have to be purchased periodically as required.

(3) As *Re-educational Therapy* avails of both craft and recreational procedures, apart from the provision of a few special items of equipment, such as a gong with striker, its requirements are covered in the two other sections of the treatment, as outlined.

The foregoing fairly exhaustive lists of requirements in both equipment and materials clearly indicate the comprehensive nature of the purchases involved in stocking and maintaining a fully developed scheme of occupational therapy, and explain the necessity for adopting sound commercial principles in dealing with the matter. This latter is the normal viewpoint in the development and management of any modern, up-to-date production plant. Here, sound business methods in both buying and selling are combined with efficient and sufficient staffing to battle successfully in the competitive war of industry. Percentage production profits will be substantially influenced by keenness in buying and selling and only those concerns whose business systems are based on modern progressive lines will survive the conflict. Without in any way detracting from the primary therapeutic purpose of an occupational therapy department, its complete development may be likened to a medley of minor production plants, composed of the various crafts in progress. Each constituent occupation involves the purchase of suitable equipment, subsequent provision of a constant supply of materials and the successful disposal of the resultant products. The diverse nature of the different crafts involved, embracing a range of widely differing activities, renders their development analogous to the theoretical fusion and centralisation, on adjacent ground, of a number of separately owned industrial factories. The complex problems, clerical and commercial, arising from such a theoretical amalgamation would give some indication of the economic difficulties to be encountered in the commercial development of occupational therapy and the necessity for rigid observance of the sound business methods associated with successful external manufacturing concerns.

*Sales*

The question of the disposal of the finished products, completed in the different sections of the occupational therapy department, raises a most important economic problem, the implications and difficulties of which will depend on environmental conditions and local circumstances peculiar to each individual hospital. Those situated within or in the vicinity of city boundaries possess advantages not enjoyed by those in rural areas, particularly when at a considerable distance from even urban populations. But a progressive occupational therapist will arrange for a system of sales contacts and methods of production that will meet local exigencies.

The vast majority of products will be consumed internally in meeting such annual hospital requirements as baskets, brushes, mats, tweeds, blankets, and other woven and knitted articles, etc., and production in these items may be regulated to avoid any substantial surplus. This will be particularly difficult of achievement in the early stages of development or in an O.T. department whose range of occupations is very limited in number, in proportion to the size and population of the hospital. If, for instance, a hospital housing 1,000 patients is dependent on a series of approximately 8 to 10 different crafts and the occupational percentage is to be maintained at a level of from 80% to 90%, reflecting the standard normally associated with a fully developed O.T. department; then even the most resourceful occupational therapist cannot in time avoid a surplus of products, the disposal of which in many cases may create an insuperable problem. A medical superintendent of a mental hospital, in such a predicament, complained that, in one month, a small section of his O.T. department had wired and completed, from factory prepared stocks, as many toothbrushes as would meet the hospital's needs for nearly ten years. This misdirected concentration, in one of the many different forms of brushcraft activity, showed a lack of appreciation of the flexibility of this particular craft in relation to production results. The work in this important section could have been regulated, to proportion production to meet the hospital's requirements for all kinds of brushes, in addition to tooth brushes, such as scrubbing brushes, both hand and deck scrubbers, sweeping brushes of all types, clothes brushes, boot brushes, nail brushes, carpet brushes, lavatory brushes, paint and distemper brushes, etc. A regulated distribution of activity in this craft, proportioned to the hospital needs, would result in continuity of operation without individual over-production.

The introduction of a wide range of occupations should reduce the numbers receiving treatment in the operation of each individual craft and this should, automatically, keep production within local requirements and thus obviate sales problems. This can be effected by the addition of a number of fancy crafts, even if less utilitarian in motive than those mentioned, such as leathercraft, special stitchcraft, raffiawork, toy manufacture, beadcraft, gessowork, wirecraft, special woodwork, nettingcraft, etc. The products of those and other such fancy crafts cannot be sold to the hospital to any appreciable extent and a market must be developed both (a) *internally* and (b) *externally*. (A) *Internally:* A substantial quantity may be disposed of, annually, by sale to the patients, their relatives, as well as visitors and members of the staff. This market may reach worthwhile standards if special discount terms are made available for cash sales at the hospital stores or O.T.D. sales section. It will have the special attraction for purchasers to secure articles to individual requirements. A handmade article, to one's own specification, at next to wholesale rate, and not generally so procurable elsewhere, will create a demand that should materially solve the problem of surplus production. (B) *Externally:* Sales to the hospital, staff, visitors, patients, and their relatives may absorb the entire production of many individual O.T. departments, particularly in hospitals of proportionately small populations. But, even in these cases, the expansion of occupational activities, leading to increased output, may necessitate a search, externally, for further markets. In some countries, central organisations have been established for the purchase of O.T. products and their subsequent sale to other public institutions at special rates. Such a central purchasing body may handle surplus production in commodities that are in constant demand for the normal requirements of other institutions, such as brushes, baskets, mats, tweeds, blankets, etc., but other contacts must be made to dispose of the surplus products of the different fancy crafts already referred to. The large general stores and firms in neighbouring towns and cities will provide a market for these, particularly if attractive discount terms are arranged. Personal interviews with the buyers in charge of the various departments in such stores may be necessary to secure satisfactory terms and quite often successful negotiations may be dependent on a *quid pro quo* arrangement. Many of these stores may be in a position to submit firm quotations for the hospital's routine requirements, even including many suitable materials for the O.T. department and mutual interests may pave the way for satisfactory commercial interchange.

Even if all these suggested methods, for some reason or another, fail to find a solution for the disposal of surplus O.T. products, there is always the organisation of periodic *Sales of Work*, where articles can be displayed at attractive prices, even if it becomes necessary to ticket them at next to cost. In any case, an enterprising occupational therapist, supported by an enthusiastic medical superintendent, will develop a successful system of sales, that will reduce the problem to merely one of routine and be reflected in the general success of the entire commercial arrangements of the department.

### 3.  *Records*

Recording the detailed activities of occupational therapy departments, as in all other forms of treatment, is of vast importance and must dovetail satisfactorily into the pre-existing system of hospital records and registers. Individual variations in the latter will undoubtedly present difficulties in attaining uniformity of outlook in standardisation. Nevertheless the plan, suggested here, embraces the essentials that should comprise the chief features of any comprehensive system and is discussed under two main heads (a) *Therapeutic* and (b) *Commercial*. This classification with subdivisions is charted below (Fig. 7), the Commercial Section, as in other diagrams, in dotted outlines, to distinguish it from the Therapeutic Sections outlined in black.

(a) *Therapeutic Records*, dealing solely with the clinical or treatment side, as distinct from those giving the commercial and accountancy details, are dealt with here, partly for convenience and because both possess a statistical relationship.

Therapeutic Records are subdivided into (1) *Individual* or *Medical Prescription Cards* and (2) *Collective*, which deal with group and sectional activities.

(1) *The Prescription Card* (Figs. 8 and 9, Pages 133, 134) may be regarded as the patient's admission ticket to occupational therapy and is completed by the appropriate medical officer. Each card contains, on one side (Fig. 8), vital information on the intellectual, emotional and conational traits of the

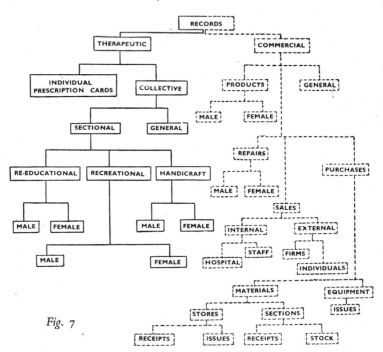

*Fig. 7*

KILLARNEY MENTAL HOSPITAL

OCCUPATIONAL THERAPY DEPT.

PRESCRIPTION CARD

Name ..................................................

Address ..................................................

No. ..................................................

Date ..................................................

Ward ..................................................

Admission Date.................. Diagnosis.................. Grade.................. Age..................

Previous Vocation.................. Previous Education.................. Previous Interests..................

Cognitional Content (*Intelligence, Memory, Understanding, Attention, etc.*)..................................................

..................................................

Emotional Content (*Hilarious, Elated, Noisy, Agitated, Depressed, Apathetic, etc.*)..................

..................................................

Conational Tendencies (*Impulses, Suicide, Escape, etc.*)..................................................

..................................................

SPECIAL RECOMMENDATIONS

(1) Handicraft Therapy..................................................

..................................................

(2) Recreational Therapy..................................................

..................................................

(3) Re-educational Therapy..................................................

..................................................

Transfers                    Date

..................................................

Signed.................................................Medical Officer

..................................................

*Fig.* 8

OCCUPATIONAL THERAPY

## PROGRESS REPORT

| | |
|---|---|
| Date....... Section....... Craft...... | Date....... Section........ Craft...... |
| Result ................................ | Result ................................ |
| .................................... | .................................... |
| Recommendation ..................... | Recommendation ..................... |
| .................................... | .................................... |
| Weight....... Signed.................. | Weight....... Signed.................. |
| Date....... Section........ Craft...... | Date....... Section........ Craft...... |
| Result ................................ | Result ................................ |
| .................................... | .................................... |
| Recommendation ..................... | Recommendation ..................... |
| .................................... | .................................... |
| Weight....... Signed.................. | Weight....... Signed.................. |
| Date....... Section........ Craft...... | Date....... Section........ Craft...... |
| Result ................................ | Result ................................ |
| .................................... | .................................... |
| Recommendation ..................... | Recommendation ..................... |
| .................................... | .................................... |
| Weight....... Signed.................. | Weight....... Signed.................. |
| Date....... Section........ Craft...... | Date....... Section........ Craft...... |
| Result ................................ | Result ................................ |
| .................................... | .................................... |
| Recommendation ..................... | Recommendation ..................... |
| .................................... | .................................... |
| Weight....... Signed.................. | Weight....... Signed.................. |
| Date....... Section........ Craft...... | Date....... Section........ Craft...... |
| Result ................................ | Result ................................ |
| .................................... | .................................... |
| Recommendation ..................... | Recommendation ..................... |
| .................................... | .................................... |
| Weight....... Signed.................. | Weight....... Signed.................. |
| Date....... Section........ Craft...... | Date....... Section........ Craft...... |
| Result ................................ | Result ................................ |
| .................................... | .................................... |
| Recommendation ..................... | Recommendation ..................... |
| .................................... | .................................... |
| Weight....... Signed.................. | Weight....... Signed.................. |

*Fig.* 9

patient introduced for treatment and is of a size suitable for filing. In addition to the usual routine information, giving age, diagnosis, grouping, etc., it carries the medical officer's recommendations with regard to the handicraft, recreational or re-educational requirements. On the reverse side (Fig. 9), provision is made for periodic reports on the patient's progress while under treatment. These reports may be weekly for a short period and then monthly or quarterly and are completed by the occupational therapist in charge of the section concerned.

These Prescription Cards may be printed in the appropriate handicraft therapy section and in different colours, based on the grading of the patients or on the sectional requirements. Thus Grade I patients may be prescribed for on Pink Cards, Green for Grade II and Blue or other colour for Grade III. Alternatively, Blue Cards may be used for the re-educational section, green cards for the recreational section, while other colours, such as pink, buff, orange, lemon, etc., for the different divisions of the handicraft section. This colour scheme of classification is merely suggested and not recommended as the proposed standard practice. It may be sufficient to meet local needs by using a different colour card as between the male and female sides of the hospital.

The prescription card, as outlined above, is for psychiatric practice and will obviously require re-drafting to suit the special adaptations of occupational therapy in other types of hospitals. In dealing with tubercular, orthopaedic, cardiac and other physical ailments, the tabulation of the mental and physical traits and tendencies in the prescription card will be subordinate to the charting of the special physical defects and requirements, with other appropriate additions and recisions. No alteration will be necessary on the reverse side of the card, as this method of progress-reporting is recommended for use in every adaptation of the treatment, both mental and physical.

(2) *Collective Records* include all those dealing with group and sectional activities and are discussed under two heads, (a) *General* and (b) *Sectional*. The former would include the weekly, monthly or annual reports of the general activities

Chief Occupational Nurse .............................................................................

....................................................... In Charge.

*Fig.* 13

KILLARNEY MENTAL HOSPITAL
OCCUPATIONAL THERAPY DEPT.
FEMALE AND MALE RE-EDUCATIONAL THERAPY SECTION.

Date................................................

Chief Re-Educational Th. Nurse.................................

### List of Class Members.

| NAME AND ADDRESS | WARD | DATE OF ADMISSION | DATE OF JOINING | AGE | PROGRESS |
|---|---|---|---|---|---|
| 1. | | | | | |
| 2. | | | | | |
| 3. | | | | | |
| 4. | | | | | |
| 5. | | | | | |
| 6. | | | | | |
| 7. | | | | | |
| 8. | | | | | |
| 9. | | | | | |
| 10. | | | | | |
| 11. | | | | | |
| 12. | | | | | |
| 13. | | | | | |
| 14. | | | | | |

### DETAILS OF PROGRESS.

| Pr. No. | |
|---|---|
| 1. | |
| 2. | |
| 3. | |
| 4. | |
| 5. | |
| 6. | |
| 7. | |
| 8. | |
| 9. | |
| 10. | |
| 11. | |
| 12. | |
| 13. | |
| 14. | |
| 15. | |

### Daily Schedule Report.

8 a.m.   TOILET, ETC. :—
9 a.m.   BREAKFAST :—
10 a.m.   TOILET :—
10.30 a.m.   RECREATIONAL THERAPY :—
12.30 p.m.   REST — TOILET :—
1 p.m.   DINNER :—
1.30 p.m.   RELAXATION :—
2.30 p.m.   TOILET :—
2.45 p.m.   HANDICRAFT THERAPY :—
4 p.m.   TOILET — AFTERNOON TEA :—
4.30 p.m.   RECREATIONAL THERAPY :—

**Evening Duty Schedule.**

3.45 p.m.   TOILET :—
6 p.m.   SUPPER :—
6.30 p.m.   RELAXATION :—
6.45 p.m.   RECREATIONAL THERAPY :—
8.15 p.m.   TOILET :—

Signed...................................... Eve. Duty Nurse.

**Night Duty Schedule.**

11.30 p.m.   TOILET :—
2 a.m.   TOILET :—
4.30 a.m.   TOILET :—
6.30 a.m.   TOILET :—

Signed...................................... Night Duty Nurse.

Signed...................................... Res. Med. Supt.

KILLARNEY MENTAL HOSPITAL.

MALE HANDICRAFT THERAPY SECTION.

## PRODUCTS WEEKLY REPORT BOOK.

Week ending ......................................................, Chief H.T. Nurse.

| Date | NAME OF PRODUCT. | Identity No. | Section | Value. | DETAILS. | Date of Sale. |
|---|---|---|---|---|---|---|
| | | | | | | |
| | | | | | | |
| | | | | | | |

Signed,......................................

Res. Med. Supt.

*Fig.* 14

KILLARNEY MENTAL HOSPITAL.
MALE HANDICRAFT SECTION.

## REPAIRS REPORT BOOK.

| Date | Section | DETAILS. | Materials Used. | Value. |
|------|---------|----------|-----------------|--------|
|      |         |          |                 |        |
|      |         |          |                 |        |
|      |         |          |                 |        |
|      |         |          |                 |        |
|      |         |          |                 |        |
|      |         |          |                 |        |
|      |         |          |                 |        |
|      |         |          |                 |        |
|      |         |          |                 |        |
|      |         |          |                 |        |
|      |         |          |                 |        |
|      |         |          |                 |        |
|      |         |          |                 |        |
|      |         |          |                 |        |
|      |         |          |                 |        |
|      |         |          |                 |        |
|      |         |          |                 |        |
|      |         |          |                 |        |
|      |         |          |                 |        |
|      |         |          |                 |        |

Date..................................

Signed, ........................................, Chief H.T. Nurse.

Signed, ...................................................

Res. Med. Supt.

*Fig.* 15

*Fig.* 16

## KILLARNEY MENTAL HOSPITAL.

### OCCUPATIONAL THERAPY DEPT.— GENERAL FINANCIAL STATEMENT.

For the Financial Year ended _____ 19___

STATEMENT OF RECEIPTS

CASH SALES

Non-Cash Sales to Hospital { Products ... ...
Repairs ... ... ...

Unsold Products—Value of Materials to Making ...

Value of Materials on Hands on_____

TOTAL RECEIPTS ...

Loss for the Year_____

RECONCILED TOTALS ...

STATEMENT OF EXPENDITURE

Value of Materials on Hands on_____

Gross Expenditure for the year ... ...

Less Cost of Equipment ... ... ...

Cost of Materials ... ... ...

TOTAL EXPENDITURE ...

PROFIT FOR THE YEAR ...

Chief Occupational Therapist_____

Storekeeper_____

Clerk_____

Resident Medical Superintendent

Dated_____

of the occupational therapy department as a whole, giving the O.T. percentage and other relevant statistics of therapeutic importance. These would be presented by the chief occupational therapist to the medical superintendent and would provide the material for the salient points to be recorded in the superintendent's annual report to his committee of management or board of governors. (b) *The Sectional Records* constitute the daily reports made regarding the activities of each section of the treatment, namely (1) *The Handicraft Section*, (2) *The Recreational Section* and (3) *The Re-educational Section*. Somewhat similar, though separate, report books in each of the three (Figs. 10-13, pp. 136-7), are in use for both the male and female sides of the hospital and each are signed by the occupational therapist or chief nurse in charge of his or her respective section. All these daily reports provide the detailed material from which the chief occupational therapist completes his general report.

This exhaustive system of therapeutic records is recommended for standard adoption, as covering the essential details of all the therapeutic sections of O.T. It presents these mainly in book form as permanent records of each day's treatment details. Prescriptions are issued in card form of suitable dimensions to facilitate filing with ease of accessibility for reference purposes. Each hospital may find it necessary to make minor adjustments in some or even all of these record forms to meet local requirements, but this is easily achieved without altering fundamentals.

(b) *Commercial Records* refer exclusively to the business side of occupational therapy and cover the accountancy, secretarial and other commercial details of the treatment. They constitute, in the main, the system of book-keeping, recommended for use. As already pointed out, the adoption of any method of commercial recording must be satisfactorily adopted to the pre-existing system of hospital accountancy in use, which latter is generally governed by statute or by a special code of hospital regulations. This will generally obviate the necessity of operating special bank or other accounts, which would simply tend to render matters more complicated and difficult for the clerical staff concerned and might easily lead to unnecessary duplication.

All cash receipts can therefore be entered into the usual hospital cash receipt book and can merely be distinguished from all other receipts by stamping in red the letters 'O.T.D.' across the block of the cash receipt book and thus permit of their being subsequently entered under their own special heading in the hospital's usual statement of receipt book. Likewise, duly vouched O.T.D. invoices can be certified for payment in bulk with all other monthly or weekly bills and likewise paid for through the hospital general account. Their classification, as such, in the general statement of expenditure book, may be facilitated by counter-signing, in red, each bill presented, with the letters 'O.T.D.'

It will, then, be only necessary, for record and stock purposes, to introduce a set of books governing (1) *Products Made*, (2) *Repairs*, (3) *Purchases*, (4) *Sales* and (5) *General Financial Statement Book*, as charted on pp. 138, 140 (Figs. 14-16).

(1) *Products:* This refers to a special report book, one each for the male and female side of the hospital, giving a weekly report of the articles made in each section (Fig. 14, Page 138), with details as to quantity and cost of materials, final costing of each article and identification number, which latter may be repeated in the appropriate sales book, on disposal of the article.

(2) *Repairs* whether revenue producing, as in the case of those executed apart from hospital requirements, or merely estimated, as in the latter case, must be recorded in a special report book (Fig. 15, p. 139). Similar to the products report book, the former gives details as to the quantity and cost of materials used and the section concerned, with date of completion of repair. Such a record, owing to the extensive quantity of repair work executed in the various sections, is absolutely essential to facilitate the production of a profit and loss account for each financial year.

(3) *Purchases:* The materials and items of equipment purchased each year should be recorded in detail in two special ledgers, one for materials and one for equipment.

These need not be specially printed, as the recording can be done in stock ledger account books of suitable size and binding procurable in any stationery stores. Likewise, similar ledgers may be used by the stores staff to record the issues of materials and equipment to the various sections of the O.T. department. The chief occupational therapist will also keep a record of the receipt of such materials and equipment from the stores and will be responsible for the production of monthly stock sheets, copies of which will be filed in the hospital stores. This will enable the head store-keeper and chief occupational therapist to keep a correct and accurate check on the receipt, distribution, use and final disposal of every item of equipment and consignment of materials. Abuses by unnecessary wastage, as well as carelessness in handling, involving unjustifiable loss, may be very readily traced by speedy investigation of these records. This will facilitate correct allocation of responsibility and tend to prevent recurrences, which might, otherwise, remain undetected. A special ledger may also be used by the stores staff to record receipt of finished articles, with identification number of each article as given in the O.T.D. products book, and space reserved to give date of sale and name of purchaser, etc.

(4) *Sales:* The recording of sales may follow the normal business practice of a general day book system of entries, with subsequent transfer to appropriate account ledgers, so necessary to record the various credit sales, which become inevitable in commercial transactions with the various general stores and outside firms, as well as individual purchasers, who have been introduced to the sales department by members of the staff. Such a system of credit facilities, if limited to strictly defined periods, does not materially add to the accountancy work, while extending the range of product disposal, and thus helps to solve what is regarded by many as one of the major problems in O.T. activities.

The number of ledger account books required for use will be dependent on the extent of credit sales permitted. One large book, indexed A-Z may be sufficient, but it makes for convenience and ease of accessibility to reserve one ledger for all transactions with the various business shops, stores, and outside firms, while credit accounts of individuals, including members of the staff, may be recorded in a separate account book, similarly indexed. This will have the further advantage of facilitating the issue of monthly statements in the case of the former, while quarterly statements may suffice in the latter owing to the comparatively smaller amounts concerned in these individual accounts and the less frequent nature of the purchases. It will be necessary in all such sales to issue detailed invoices, giving date and method of dispatch, when the goods are not taken delivery of directly by the purchaser. Copies of these invoices will be filed as record of dispatch. In the case of goods sent per rail, a special goods dispatch book, giving details of each consignment, is required to secure the signature of the local railway official certifying receipt in good condition and recording cost of carriage, etc. The necessity for this becomes obvious in case of damage in transit or failure to reach proper destination or within the scheduled time. It also provides a permanent record of the amount of carriage on each individual consignment, and thus permits the inclusion of this charge on the invoice for posting on the same date, where cost of transport is debited against purchaser's account by pre-arrangement.

In connection with the sales of finished products to the hospital, as distinct from repairs effected, which is dealt with in the special repairs report book, already referred to, a special ledger account book must be utilised for recording such non-cash transactions. This will give the details of the products bought by the hospital, with date of sale and estimated cost in each case. This latter figure will be based on the actual cost of such products, if procured from outside sources, and will be determined by securing written quotations where a fixed contract price is not otherwise available. While the actual expenditure involved, on the part of the hospital, in these items is confined to the cost of the materials of manufacture, the difference between the latter and the prevailing commercial value of the finished product represents an important saving, which materially influences the profit and loss account figures for each financial year. The entries made in this ledger will, therefore, facilitate the immediate preparation of the latter account, by obviating last-minute calculations, that have already been made through the method of periodic recording.

(5) *General Financial Statement Book:* This book may be specially printed on the lines of the usual hospital General Summary of Accounts Book, with the appropriate arrangement of headings (as in Fig. 16, p. 140) giving for each year, the total amount of receipts, both (a) *Cash*, as taken from the hospital statement of receipts book, and (b) *Non-Cash*, as recorded in detail in the special report books already referred to. Provision is, likewise, made for a statement of the total annual amount expended in the purchase of both materials and equipment. It will differ from the hospital summary of accounts book, in that it will give an annual general statement of accounts for the entire O.T. department, incorporating a profit and loss account for each completed financial year.

It will, therefore, record for each year the total receipts, both actual cash and estimated as in the case of sales to the hospital and repairs executed for the hospital, which latter figures will be summarised from the special report books dealing with these items. These receipts will be offset, on the next page facing, by the details of the expenditure on materials and equipment for the corresponding year. By a system crediting on the receipts side the actual value of the unused materials and finished products on hands at the end of the year and debiting on the expenditure side the actual value of the unused materials and finished products on hands at the commencement of the year, a record of the profit or loss on the general working of the O.T. department is thus available. It will be noted, therefore, that this report book gives merely a summarised account of the receipts and expenditure, to effect its primary purpose of estimating the profit or loss for any particular year under review. Its annual preparation involves the co-operation and mutual assistance of the occupational therapists, the stores and clerical staffs of the hospital and is submitted for the approval of the medical superintendent over the signature of the chief occupational therapist, the chief clerk and storekeeper.

Associated with the work of accountancy recording and equally important is the essential volume of secretarial work, including both (a) *Writing* and (b) *Filing*. These constitute the main connecting link between the O.T. department's internal and external interests. They are in effect the central exchange, providing communication between the O.T.D. supplies and sales sections with both its many suppliers and various purchasers. The operators are drawn from the clerical and stores staff of the hospital, with the chief clerk, storekeeper and chief occupational therapist as supervisors under the medical superintendent as chief supervisor. All assume appropriate conjoint responsibility in the smooth working of this so-called exchange.

(a) *Writing:* The purchasing of materials and equipment will involve a good deal of correspondence both in the initial inquiry stages and the subsequent placing of definite orders. This will be very substantially supplemented by the volume of secretarial work in making sales contacts and invoicing and dispatching purchased products. The greater part of this work will be carried out by the hospital clerical staff, under the guidance and supervision of the chief occupational therapist, the clerk and storekeeper, whose staffs will have the additional work of recording the entries in the various ledgers and report books previously referred to.

(b) *Filing:* As an immediate concomitant of most of the secretarial work will arise the necessity of filing the various letters to facilitate speedy handling of the daily items requiring attention. The system of filing adopted may vary according to personal tastes, but it is considered advisable to take separate files for each item of equipment and each type of material required for any individual occupation, as distinct from filing each supplier in separate folders. Separate filing compartments should be used for materials and equipment, while sales and accounts files will be based on the more usual individual system, to facilitate book-keeping and accountancy.

It will be realised from a detailed analysis of the foregoing that the position of the commercial side of occupational therapy has not been over-stated or unduly magnified. The success of the entire departments will, in no small way, be dependent on the efficacy of the commercial principles adopted. Simplicity, combined with thoroughness, must form the chief features of the economic methods used, to ensure their smooth incorporation into the pre-existing system of hospital accountancy, without unduly adding to or complicating the volume of clerical work already involved. Methods of buying and selling must also be based on modern, accepted standards, to prevent loss on outlay, without in any way minimising the primary importance of the therapeutic element of the treatment, which is the paramount consideration.

# CHAPTER XI.

## PSYCHOLOGICAL ANALYSIS

### MENTAL DISEASES

CRAFT ANALYSIS, which provides for a detailed classification and investigation of the various occupations suitable for treatment, does not exceed in importance the necessity for a corresponding analysis of the different mental diseases and mental states requiring occupational treatment. This classification and study of abnormal mental conditions is described as psychological analysis and is essential for the complete and scientific administration of occupational therapy in all its branches and divisions. No rational application of occupational treatment is possible in the absence of a full and proper understanding of the different types of patient material submitted for treatment. Just as the medical member of the staff in charge of an O.T. section must be conversant with the details and qualities of the different crafts, to enable him to complete a prescription card, competently, so likewise the therapist in charge of an occupational section must have an intelligent appreciation of at least the different mental states, in the absence of a detailed knowledge of the various mental diseases proper.

An exhaustive psychological analysis, therefore, from the O.T. point of view will investigate and discuss not only (a) *Individual Mental Diseases*, but also (b) *Mental States* or *Symptoms*, including the different *mental types*. The Mental States or Symptoms are simply the prominent and observed features of the former and will, consequently, vary in relation not alone to the disease itself, but also to the progress in each individual disease. For instance the motor excitement associated with the Katatonic form of Schizophrenia may be replaced by a condition of inertia (pseudo-depression) in the course of the disease and either of these two mental states may exhibit characteristic differences from the corresponding states occurring in the Manic-Depressive Psychosis. The recognition and proper apprec-

148

iation of these differences are essential in providing the correct therapeutic procedure in any individual case.

(A) *Mental Diseases:* Owing to the great variety of mental diseases and the differences in the symptomatology of each, as exhibited in individual cases, it is not possible to give a purely logical definition of Insanity. It has been described as a Perversion of the Ego. As the Ego is a very variable quantity and not easily reduced to a common denominator for comparative purposes, such a terse description is obviously unsatisfactory. Of the many definitions propounded by various authorities, perhaps that given by the late Dr. Maudsley, London, is worth recording. In Maudsley's *Pathology of Mind* he states:

'By insanity of mind is meant such derangement of the leading functions of thought, feeling and will, together or separately, as disables the person from thinking the thoughts, feeling the feelings and doing the duties of the social body in, for, and by which he lives.'

This definition covers the three main activities of the mind: (1) *Cognition* (intellectual function), (2) *Affect* (emotional activity) and (3) *Conation* (concerning behaviour and conduct).

The classifications of mental diseases, in the absence of a common generally approved basis, are many and varied and each has had to be altered from time to time to keep up with current advances and altered outlook consequent on scientific progress and development, particularly during the past thirty years. The introduction of psycho-analysis and the various new physical treatments, not least among which is included occupational therapy, has created a more hopeful and rational attitude towards prognosis in psychological medicine generally. The gradual development of this scientific and more practical outlook on mental disease has caused radical alterations in the different classifications, and these changes have extended to the designations of many individual mental diseases. For instance, the unsatisfactory title *Dementia Praecox*, elaborated by Kraepelin, was changed in 1908 by Bleuler into the now universally accepted term *Schizophrenia*.

The difficulty in standard classification is also intensified by the diversity of viewpoint regarding the causal factors. Those diseases of definite somatic origin, such as General Paresis, Toxic Psychoses, Senile Psychoses, etc., are more readily amenable to classification than those where the absolute causative factor is either doubtful or unknown. This difficulty is also aggravated by the fact that the mind, though often exhibiting disease in part, reacts as a whole and the consequent disharmony between the various activities cannot be viewed exclusively in the light of individual morbid processes. In such cases the individual reactions and adjustments, though often following a general pattern, may be subject to the personal differences arising from the varying factors associated with personality make-up as well as unduplicated environmental influences. In other words the importance of treating the individual patient, rather than the psychosis as diagnosed, creates individual differences in viewpoint, which add to the difficulties of classification.

For these reasons, failure to strike a generally accepted common basis for classification has resulted in a multiplicity of groupings as numerous as the different bases adopted. It has, in fact, been a case of *Quot homines tot sententiae.* A classification by Kraepelin, meeting with wide approval, has been based on the symptoms exhibited by each psychosis, while a more generally favoured arrangement by Meyer, regarded mental diseases as different types of reaction.

The British Royal Medico-Psychological Association in 1933 approved of the following official classification, representing clinical pictures of types of mental disorder, with which all psychiatrists are familiar:—

(A)  *Oligophrenia* (Amentia, Mental Deficiency).
    (a)  Idiocy.
    (b)  Imbecility.
    (c)  Feeblemindedness (Moron).
    (d)  Moral Deficiency.

(B)  *Neuroses and Psychoneuroses.*
    (a)  Exhaustion States (including Neurasthenia).
    (b)  Anxiety States.
    (c)  Compulsions, Obsessions and Phobias.

(d) Hysteria.

(e) Mixed and other forms.

(C) *Schizophrenic Psychoses.*

    (a) Dementia Praecox.

        (i) Simple.

        (ii) Hebephrenic.

        (iii) Katatonic.

        (iv) Paranoid.

    (b) Paraphrenia.

    (c) Other Forms.

(D) *Psychopathic Constitution* (including Paranoia).

(E) *Affective Psychoses.*

    (a) Manic-Depressive Psychosis (Cyclothymia).

        (i) Elation.

        (ii) Depression.

        (iii) Stupor.

    (b) Involutional Melancholia.

(F) *Confusional States.*

(G) *Epileptic Psychoses.*

(H) *General Paralysis.*

(I) *Other Psychoses associated with Organic Brain Disease.*

(K) *Undetermined Types.*

The above classification does not appear to lay any emphasis on such well-recognised clinical entities as the Traumatic Psychoses, Senile Psychoses and Alcoholic Psychoses, though these are referred to in a special Part II Section, dealing with aetiological factors. The compact nature of the classification, however, is a very commendable feature.

Kraepelin's symptomatological classification was, with certain modifications, including Bleuler's alterations, adopted by the American Psychiatric Association in 1934. This classification is both descriptive in character and exhaustive in its wide scope. Symptom-grouping, too, has a special significance for occupational purposes, as it tends to simplify the distribution and apportioning of patient material in relation to available occupations. Mainly for these reasons, the modified Kraepelinian classification, listed as follows, will be observed in this text, making appropriate alterations in the original order of grouping to suit analysis for O.T. purposes.

1. Schizophrenic Psychoses.
2. Manic-Depressive Psychoses.
3. Paranoic Psychoses.
4. Senile Psychoses.
5. Involutional Psychoses.
6. Epileptic Psychoses.
7. Alcoholic Psychoses.
8. Syphilitic Psychoses.
9. Psychoneuroses.
10. Psychoses with Mental Deficiency (Amentia).
11. Psychoses due to drugs or exogenous poisons.
12. Psychoses with Infectious Diseases (Meningitis, Acute Chorea, etc.), (including Epidemic Encephalitis).
13. Traumatic Psychoses.
14. Psychoses due to new growth.
15. Psychoses associated with organic changes in the nervous system. (Multiple Sclerosis, Paralysis Agitans, Huntington's Chorea, Tabes Dorsalis).
16. Psychoses associated with disturbances of circulation.
17. Psychoses due to Metabolic diseases.
18. Psychoses with psychopathic personality.

It is not feasible in an occupational therapy textbook to discuss in detail all the eighteen types listed above—some of which include further classification into widely differing clinical entities, though grouped under one heading. In actual practice the first nine compose the vast majority of psychotic conditions, met with it in the public mental hospitals. No. 10—Mental Deficiency (Amentia) conditions are generally treated exclusively in special institutions. Of these nine conditions, the Schizophrenic group, from the occupational therapy point of view, is the most important, particularly owing to the relatively higher numbers requiring occupational treatment. Although the admissions of schizophrenic psychotics to public mental hospitals constitute only 15% to 20% of the annual total, the resident numbers reach 60% to 70% of all cases, owing to the progressive nature of the disease and the tendency to chronicity. The second group—the Manic-Depressive Psychotics—are almost of equal importance as they constitute a first admission percentage which often exceeds that of Schizophrenia—in some cases reaching as high as 50%. Their relative importance, however, is offset by the very much lower resident percentage owing to the generally favourable and often short course in the disease.

The remaining six (Nos. 3-9) in this grouping, although of relatively lower admission percentages, require equal consideration, from the point of view of O.T. analysis, as those of the first two groups. Group 10, dealing with Amentia (Oligophrenia or Mental Deficiency), necessitates a specialised application of occupational treatment, where the therapeutic element has to be made subservient to the vocational aspect. For this reason, chiefly, it is not proposed to submit Mental Deficiency conditions to psychological analysis here, as this would be more appropriately covered in a special O.T. treatise dealing solely with Amentia (Oligophrenia).

The remaining groups 11 to 18 will be dealt with, in accordance with the nature of the special symptoms arising in each, as these latter may not be covered in the analysis of the other psychoses, due regard, however, being paid to their suitability for O.T. application.

Group 1                    *Schizophrenia*

This is a disease mainly of the adolescent or growing period and, because of the diversity and variable nature of its symptomatology, raises O.T. problems as difficult as they are numerous. Four main clinical varieties are described, all exhibiting in common an emotional dulling or mental apathy so universally characteristic of the disease, namely: (A) Simplex type, (B) Katatonia, (C) the Paranoid type and (D) Hebephrenic type. Although each type exhibits certain distinguishing features, one must not overlook the possibility of one type passing into the other in the generally prolonged course of the disease. An additional characteristic, common to all types, excluding the Simplex type, is the presence of both delusions and hallucinations, and this duad of symptoms, arising from the disorders of reasoning and of the senses, shows characteristic differences in the three clinical types mentioned. The general mental apathy present in all forms of the disease arises from disturbances of the emotional side, as already detailed in the chapter dealing with Re-educational Therapy, namely *Athymia* or loss of emotion and *Parathymia* or distorted emotion. This emotional indifference typifies the withdrawal from the external world into one of phantasy and day-dreaming, confirming the introverted nature of all schizophrenics. Failure of normal extroversion is a prominent feature of the disease and O.T. assumes a most important role in its restoration.

(A) *Simplex Type*. This type shows the general apathy and lack of personal concern, so prominent a feature of the psychosis. The emotional disturbances leading to loss of ambition and a state of disinterestedness emphasise the introverted nature of the personality change. Judgment, particularly regarding moral values, shows alteration, though delusions are very rarely in evidence. This absence of delusions, as well as hallucinations, distinguishes the simple from the three other clinical types. Because of the personality changes and defective judgment conduct becomes abnormal and the natural interest in self-advancement, education and occupation is gradually lost, leading to moodiness and indolency and not rarely to vagrancy and delinquency.

(B) *Katatonia*. In the older schools of psychiatry, this has been described rather erroneously, though persistently, as consisting of alternating states of (1) Excitement, (2) Stupor and (3) Depression. In our view there is no true stupor in Katatonia, merely a pseudo-stupor in which the immobility and mutism present, give a false impression of stupor, as well as of depression. The word 'stupor,' derived from the Latin *stupere*, meaning to stun, refers to the stunning or dulling of the senses or mental faculties, which characterises stupor. That such dulling does not occur in the pseudo-stupor of Katatonia is described in detail further on. Likewise, an absolute or true depression is not seen in the disease. Any depression described is only of a relative nature and is merely confused with the state of mental indifference and poverty of emotion so pronounced in Schizophrenia. The disorders of emotion occurring in the disease are of such a nature as not to permit of a genuine depressive reaction.

For these reasons Katatonia might more accurately be divided into three distinct phases, which have a tendency to show irregular alternation, namely, (1) *The Active Stage*, (2) *The Stage of Inertia* and (3) *The Quiescent Stage*. (1) The *Active Stage* is characterised by a variety of symptoms, chief of which include *Motor Excitement, Mannerisms, Stereotypies, impulsive and destructive behaviour* and may last for many days or even only hours at a time. The *Stereotypies* may take the form of *Echopraxia*—imitating movements of others in the immediate vicinity—or *Echolalia*—repeating words or phrases spoken by others nearby. A special form of speech stereotypy, known as *Verbigeration*, consists of the continuous repetition of some word or series of words, often lasting for lengthy periods. *Echolalia* and *Echopraxia* are examples of *automatic obedience* of an active type. This latter is a condition of pathological suggestibility where external commands may be carried out in a blind automatic manner, regardless of their absurdity or the possible dangers involved in their execution. *Mannerisms* are also special forms of stereotyped movements, such as grimacing, tic-like movements, as well as peculiarities of gait and gestures. Many of these forms of active and impulsive behaviour may result from hallucinations of sight or hearing and quite often the sudden nature of their oncoming, not excluding their possible homicidal or suicidal content, call for the strict and unremitting attention of the O.T. personnel dealing with such patients. (2) *The Stage of Inertia* or *the passive phase* of Katatonia, inaccurately described as stupor and depression, is a well recognised clinical entity, characterised by a state of inactivity or immobility, in which *Negativism* is a very prominent feature. This consists of an attitude of resistiveness and refusal to accede to any requests made, even those in the patient's own interest. It is reflected in the patient's refusal of food and a condition of self-imposed silence known as

*Mutism.* Negativism, in the active phase, is shown by the tendency to do the exact opposite to that required. In the inertia stage of Katatonia, a passive form of *automatic obedience* known as *flexibilitas cerea* (waxy flexibility) may be demonstrated. In this condition a patient may remain for even lengthy periods in any unusual or uncomfortable position, when so placed by others. The limbs may be moulded, as it were, into any special position, assuming a wax-like rigidity.

Patients in Katatonic Inertia remain often with unclosed eyes, in a state of immobility and assume a mask-like appearance and condition of complete indifference to either surroundings or personal requirements. Saliva is retained, often with drooling, food is refused, necessitating artificial feeding and no attention is paid to the needs of personal cleanliness or dressing. Notwithstanding this picture of apparent total and complete apathy, visual and aural sensory impressions are strongly registered and most patients returning to the active or quiescent state may recount, often with embarassing effects, many of the conversations or incidents occurring in the immediate vicinity during this stage of inertia.

(3) *The Quiescent* form of Katatonia may be described as the period of remission or intermission of the more usual symptoms, which intervenes between active phases of the disease or between alternating attacks of inertia and excitement. These periods of remission may be seen in the other clinical types of Schizophrenia, but are of much more frequent occurrence in Katatonia. During these remissions, patients adjust themselves very closely to normal requirements, even under home conditions. Nothing contributes more to the prolongation of these remission periods or tends to increase their frequency than occupational therapy under appropriate prescription.

(C) *The Paranoid Type* is so called because of a certain symptomatological similarity to what is described as True Paranoia (Paranoia-ides—identical with or similar to Paranoia). The similarity is based on the fact that both conditions are mainly characterised by delusions of persecution. In the paranoid type, however, these delusions are not fixed or systematised, being bizarre, illogical and changeable and they are further complicated by associated hallucinations, as well as the accompanying schizoid picture of emotional impairment and general maladjustment. This maladjustment, influenced by the fantastic delusions present as well as the hallucinations, may be represented by sudden and erratic behaviour. In some cases the delusions may be more of the expansive or hypochondriacal type, but the fleeting nature of the delusional content may lead the psychosis to assume katatonic or hebephrenic trends. Just as the prognosis of the paranoid type is the least favourable so does it cause greater O.T. difficulties in both prescription and administration. The gross disturbance of the auto-critical faculty, with its associated loss of insight, creates difficulties in securing sufficient contact to assess therapeutic requirements, as well as maintaining rapport in the treatment prescribed.

(D) *Hebephrenia.* This type is distinguished from the other clinical types by the extreme nature of the introversion present, leading to a marked tendency towards seclusion. This seclusiveness is further reinforced, in a large number of cases, by a pronounced inaccessibility, showing the extreme regressive nature of the condition, and is often incorrectly regarded and described as a form of depression. It is this *regression,* in which symptoms are characterised more by a negativeness than by anything of a positively demonstrable nature, which creates occupational therapy problems, that may only be resolved by re-educational measures. Occasionally the resultant disintegration of personality may be so pronounced as to defy even the most persistent attempts at re-education. The seclusiveness, however, may at times be replaced by mannerisms with silly grimacing, incoherency and senseless laughter and often emotional outbursts and excitement. These symptoms, however, would appear to indicate more a katatonic phase. Hallucinations and delusions, not always demonstrable, are present in the hebephrenic type, but they are generally of a fleeting, bizarre type. Ideas of reference have also been described in the condition, but are generally transient and any tendency towards fixity would appear to incline towards the Paranoid form of the disease.

As already mentioned, while these clinical divisions of schizophrenia have each distinguishing features, the variability in the course of the disease and the general unity in its symptomatology may show changes from one type to the other. A common characteristic of all types of the disease is the marked introversion present. The American authority, Noyes, referring to this point states:—

'In Schizophrenia we may see introversion carried to an extreme that effectually encysts the patient and prevents contacts with reality and its painful problems.'

Because of this introversion, as well as the preoccupancy of the schizoid, the prescription difficulties in craft selection become no less aggravating than the obstacles presented in securing craft contact.

### Group 2          *The Manic-Depressive Psychosis*

*The Manic-Depressive Psychosis* includes the two conditions (A) *Mania* and (B) *Melancholia*, which prior to their being thus grouped by Kraepelin in 1896 were regarded as separate mental diseases. The fact that maniacal and depressive phases may alternate in the same psychotic would appear to justify this grouping under a common head, although each phase has characteristically separate clinical features.

(A) *Mania* is classified into three main clinical types (1) *Hypomania*, (2) *Acute Mania* and (3) *Chronic Mania*. Some authorities describe a fourth type—*Delirious Mania*, but this is generally a confusional psychosis of toxic origin. All three types are characterised by a well-recognised triad of symptoms—(a) *Elation*, (b) *Flow of Ideas* and (c) *Motor Excitement*, each representing, respectively, a disorder of the affective, cognitional and conational (volitional) functions of the mind. (a) *Elation* occurs as a markedly exaggerated form of well-being—a state of exhiliration in which nothing appears impossible of either attainment or achievement. This feeling of euphoria or exaltation, often leading to delusions of grandeur, shows fluctuations of mood in keeping with the general unstableness so prominent in the disease. Inappropriate joyousness and laughter may suddenly be replaced by a display of tears equally irrelevant. Any interference with the whims and fancies of the elated patient arouses extreme anger, accompanied by a stream of verbal and often obscene abuse.

(b) *Flow of Ideas* results from overactivity in the association of ideas and these are produced with such rapidity that they over-run the normal speed of speech reproduction and hence a number of ideas fail to be expressed, the result giving an appearance of incoherency. This incoherence, however, is only relative and is not of the absolute type seen in advanced cases of Dementia.

(c) *Motor Excitement* is represented by a continuous pressure of overactivity, often to the extent of reaching an extreme state of turbulency and agressiveness of a noisy and abusive type. There is marked resentment of any limitation or restriction of movements.

In addition, there is general loss of insight, often with delusions and with a *pronounced distractibility of attention.* This failure to maintain concerted attention raises O.T. difficulties, but can be utilised with success in securing direction and control of the disturbed and fleeting thought processes by diverting the attention towards less disturbing and less objectionable activities. Every intelligent nurse recognises this facility for influencing the disturbed, over-active maniacal patient.

(1) *Hypomania* may be described as a mild form of Mania, where the symptoms of Elation, Excitement and Flow of Ideas are not developed to the extent found in the acute or other forms of Mania. The early developing stage of a maniacal phase may be of this kind and is described as a Hypomania if the symptoms persist in this mild form. Because of this less active nature of the disease, hypomaniacs are not often submitted for hospital treatment. It is only when the behaviour becomes of such an asocial character that hospitalisation is necessary.

(2) *Acute Mania* represents the disease in its most energetic form when there is complete unrestraint with regard to affect, thought processes and general psychomotor activity, as described above. This extreme, unrestricted and uncontrollable form of muscular speech and thought functioning and

general hyperactivity creates nursing problems unequalled in psychiatry. The mischievousness, destructiveness and necessity for individual attention, both with regard to food and personal cleanliness, in the fully developed acute maniac, make demands on hospital personnel that have repercussions on the tact and patience of the nursing staff as on the economic endeavours of the administration generally. Here, O.T. makes an important contribution to the solution of the multiple nature of the problem.

(3) *Chronic Mania* may be described as a persistent form of the maniacal phase, the symptoms of which, while showing mitigation in their more usual form, are, nevertheless, uninterrupted by periods of either recovery or depression. The condition occurs generally in middle or late life and quite often with a previous history of recurring maniacal attacks. The associated state of elation and excitement may persist with varying intensity for periods even as long as twenty to thirty years. Hallucinations and delusions are very rare but the mischievousness and querulousness of the acute maniac are pronounced.

(B) *Melancholia* shows four main clinical types differentiated, similarly to Mania, by the severity of the symptoms into (1) *Simple Melancholia*, (2) *Acute Melancholia*, (3) *Depressive Stupor* and (4) *Chronic Melancholia*. The acute form of the disease has been subdivided into many other types, according to the predominating symptom present, e.g. *acute agitated*, when agitation is prominent, *acute delusional*, when delusions are the emphasised feature, *acute resistive*, when there is marked resistance to attention, including refusal of food, necessitating artificial feeding, and *acute hypochondriacal*, when ideas and delusions regarding health form the chief picture. *Involutional Melancholia* and *Senile Melancholia* are also differentiated, because of the special symptomatology associated with these physiological epochs in life and are separately described.

Melancholia may occur in varying degrees in normal people, described popularly as a 'fit of the blues' or 'feeling in bad form,' but it becomes pathological when the extent of the depression present is not justified by the circumstances of the case and when complicated by loss of insight into the nature of the condition. Just as in mania, melancholia is characterised by a triad of symptoms, which are in the opposite pole to mania. These symptoms, namely (1) depression (affective), (2) difficulty in thinking (cognitional) and (3) general psychomotor retardation (conational).

(1) *The depression* present is in contrast to the elation in mania and consists of sadness, with a feeling of misery out of proportion to the circumstances present. Because of the depressive nature of the disease, all melancholics have to be rated as potential suicides and some authorities are of the opinion that this psychosis is responsible for nearly 75% of all suicides and quite often the milder the depression, the greater the tendency to suicide. This latter point must be kept well in mind in the occupational treatment of both the simple and convalescing melancholic.

(2) *Difficulty in thinking* or retardation of ideation is a marked concomitant of all forms of depression. Replies to questions are irritatingly slow and more often than not of a monosyllabic nature. This poverty of thought is in keeping with the general inertia found in the condition, as well as the lack of interest in external happenings, and even in personal appearance and personal needs.

(3) *General psychomotor retardation* is very pronounced in melancholia, in marked contradistinction to mania. There is general inertia present and all movements, following request, are slow in both initiation and execution. This inertia may be so pronounced as to necessitate assistance in dressing and undressing as well as in dealing with food and other personal needs, although there is no clouding of intellect or memory defects and no disorientation.

The melancholic, however, attempts to rationalise his general state of depression, inactivity and irresolution by giving vent to delusions. These are generally of a self-accusatory nature, but often they have a nihilistic and hypochondriacal tendency. The melancholic believes that he has committed 'the unpardonable sin' and that he 'is of no use in this life.' Hallucinations are generally very rarely met with in melancholia. Just as in Schizophrenia, however, it

should be borne in mind that the three acute forms of Melancholia may merge into each other in any individual case
and the distinction, though arbitrary, is merely of clinical
significance.

(1) *Simple Melancholia*, like Hypomania, characterises a
mild form of the disease where the depression, general
retardation and inactivity is not so pronounced as in Acute
Melancholia. In this type there may be a certain amount
of insight into the nature of the condition and delusions
are generally not prominent. Obsessions and hypochondriacal ideas may form the chief features.

(2) *Acute Melancholia* comprises the typical and more
usual form of the disease. The triad of symptoms, described
previously, are prominent features and the typical delusions,
associated with the condition, are very marked. Bleuler
stated that these delusions are mainly concerned with sin,
health or fortune, and comparing the hypochondriacal
delusions of the Schizophrenic and the Melancholic, he stated
that the Schizophrenic anxieties are chiefly concerned with
the present, while the melancholic worries about the future,
and it might be added here, also about the past. This preoccupation concerning the future and the past is of importance
from the suicidal point of view.

(3) *Depressive Stupor*, known also as *Anergic Stupor*, is
the most profound type of stupor met with. There is complete
immobility, with clouding of consciousness and no response
to external stimuli. All personal requirements are neglected—
the patient being confined to bed, wet and dirty in habits
and requiring to be tube-fed. The face is generally mask-like,
and intensely depressive delusions appear to be the sole
preoccupation.

(4) *Chronic Melancholia*. This condition, more prevalent
formerly than chronic mania, like the latter is characterised
by a persistence generally in a less intense manner of the
symptoms of the acute phase. When recovery from the
acute melancholic states does not occur after the usual six
to twelve months' course, the condition passes into a chronic
state of depression. The very favourable influence, exerted
by Electro-Convulsant Therapy, on all forms of depression,

particularly the involutional type, will tend to reverse its frequency ratio with that of chronic mania.

*Alternating states* of the Manic-Depressive Psychosis are also described, such as (a) *True Alternating*, (b) *Continuous Alternating*, (c) *Circular*, etc., but the symptoms displayed in each phase of these are identical with the acute phases as already described and require no further special analysis from the O.T. point of view.

*Group* 3        *The Paranoic Psychoses*

*The Paranoic Psychoses*, according to modern tendency, include all paranoic conditions, ranging from (1) *the Paranoid Schizophrenic* pole, on the one hand, to the other extreme, characterised by what is described as (2) *True Paranoia*. Kraepelin designated a condition intermediate between the latter two poles, which he called (3) *Paraphrenia*. (1) *Paranoid Schizophrenia* (Dementia Paranoides) has been already discussed.

(2) The word *Paranoia* is derived from the Greek words 'para' — beside and 'vous' — the mind or intellect. The Greek word 'Para' used in psychological terminology as a prefix, may more accurately be interpreted as meaning 'distorted.' Thus, Paramnesia may be defined as distorted memory and paralogia, occurring in the Ganser Syndrome and Schizophrenia, as distorted answering (in reply to simple questions). Kraepelin described Paranoia as a chronic psychosis, characterised by fixed, systematised delusions of persecution, with reasoning on all other topics, not connected with the delusional system, being unimpaired. The outstanding mental mechanism in the condition is known as *Projection*, where the psychotic's failings and motives are projected on to others and attributed to them. Three stages in the course of the disease are recognised (1) *the Stage of Suspicion*, in which simple casual events are misinterpreted and construed as having sinister and hidden meanings with a special personal reference and this leads to the development of (2) *the Stage of Persecution*, in which delusions of a persecutory nature tend to become evolved into a fixed, unalterable system. Under the influence of these delusions, the Paranoiac

rationalises the persecution of his imaginary enemies, by developing grandiose and exalted ideas. The persistent nature of his 'persecution' can only be explained on the grounds of his 'exalted rank.' This forms (3) *the Stage of Grandeur*, in which delusions of exaltation, sometimes of a religious nature, tend to dominate the picture.

Several different clinical forms of Paranoia are described, each characterising the predominant symptoms, such as (a) *Persecutory*, where delusions of persecution predominate, (b) *Querulant* or *Litigious type*, where the Paranoiac may spend his entire time in arraigning his 'persecutors,' (c) *the Religious type*, (d) *the Amorous* or *Jealous type*, (e) *the Hypochondriacal type*, where preoccupation with health forms the main picture. Kraepelin distinguished two main types—(1) *Mattoids*, embracing the many faddists and reformers who, in a characteristically isolated manner, spend their lives preaching their pet theories in public, without coming into conflict with social requirements and (2) *Egocentrics* who constitute cases of 'True' Paranoia, where the delusions are concerned with self, in contrast to the altruistic ideas of the Mattoid.

Gierlich and Friedmann described *Abortive* or *Recurrent forms* of Paranoia, where typical paranoid syndromes develop, lasting for several weeks, always ending in recovery with full insight into the nature of the disease, but with a definite tendency to recur.

Lasegue and Falret described a *communicated form of Paranoia—Folie a deux*. This condition arises in the case of two people, generally mother and daughter, or husband and wife, etc., leading a secluded existence, where the more active and dominant personality of the two with a definite paranoic psychosis, induces it in the other person, the passive and more submissive of the two. The induced condition generally disappears from the latter on separation from the dominant partner.

(3) *Paraphrenia* may be regarded broadly as a form of Paranoia, which is merely complicated by the presence of hallucinations, generally of a bizarre and absurd nature. *Neologisms* or the coining of new words is very prevalent

in the condition. Most authorities agree that a paranoic psychosis occurring in a case of a highly intellectual personality tends to run a course akin to 'True' Paranoia, without the development of hallucinations or terminal mental deterioration. Where intellectual capacity is of low grade or below average, the paranoic psychosis tends to pass ultimately into a paraphrenic phase as described. Kraepelin recognised four types of Paraphrenia, which are not easily distinguishable and of very doubtful utility in classification, namely (1) *Paraphrenia Systematica*, (2) *Paraphrenia Phantastica*, (3) *Paraphrenia Expansiva* and (4) *Paraphrenia Confabulans*.

Capgras has described a syndrome, peculiar to women, occurring in Paraphrenia, in which there occurs misidentification of persons, resulting in 'the illusion of doubles,' where the patient rationalises her failure to identify people by positing the theory of 'doubles.'

## Group 4      *The Senile Psychoses*

*The Senile Psychoses* embrace a wide range of clinical conditions, of importance from the occupational therapy point of view, particularly the *pre-senile types*. The symptoms and signs of the more usual senile dotage must be distinguished from those of *Senile Dementia*. Old age is a natural terminal condition represented by (1) *Simple deterioration*, which is characterised by a lessening of physical activity, as well as mental acuity, with loss of recent memory (anterograde amnesia) and disinterest in former social contacts. There is associated irritability and insomnia with a tendency to live in the past and failure to assimilate new experiences. These simple deteriorative changes, when of a mild form, are a natural end-result that may occur after the age of sixty, generally later, and constitute normal senile dotage. It is only when they become more pronounced with added concomitant mental changes that they pass into the stage of Senile Dementia, but there is no definite line of demarcation to indicate when this transition has taken place.

(2) *Senile Dementia* shows four types differing only according to the prominence of the prevailing mental states present, namely, (a) *Senile Mania*, (b) *Senile Melancholia*,

(c) *Senile Confused type* and (d) *Senile Paranoid type*. In (a) *Senile Mania*, there is mild elation with a noisy restlessness, accompanied by marked insomnia. The general signs and symptoms of Hypomania and sometimes of acute mania are present, but the typical 'flight of ideas' is not prominent owing to the poverty of ideation so marked in all senile dements.

(b) *Senile Melancholia* does not differ very markedly from a depressive phase of the Manic-Depressive Psychosis, excepting that the delusions are more of a hypochondriacal nature and hallucinations are more frequent.

(c) *The Senile Confused type* is more an episodic condition of senile dementia, where there is disorientation and confusion, complicated with insomnia and hallucinations. There is marked tendency towards resistiveness and restlessness, with aimless wandering and consequent danger of exhaustion.

(d) *The Senile Paranoiac* may show the more usual paranoid symptoms, but the persecutory delusions tend to be more bizarre and absurd owing to the normal senile failure of intellect and judgment.

(3) *The Presenile Psychosis* (Senium Praecox), mainly of three types (a) *Presbyophrenia*, (b) *Alzheimer's Disease* and (c) *Pick's Disease* are regarded as senile conditions, occurring prematurely (presenile) between the ages of 40 and 60. It is often difficult to differentiate between the three conditions and many authorities are inclined to dispute their separate clinical existence. All three show the more usual features of senile deterioration, but each has certain emphasised features, which probably justify their clinical separation.

(a) *Presbyophrenia* is a presenile condition, more commonly occurring in women, characterised by (1) *Paramnesia* (Pseudomnesia), distortion of memory. The presence of anterograde amnesia (loss of recent memory) and defect of retention, cause the patient to indulge in *Confabulation* (Korsakov's Syndrome), that is recalling incidents and events that have never taken place. There is also (2) *a great press of purposeless activity*, described as 'occupational delirium,' often of a destructive nature and accompanied by a marked loquaciousness (logorrhea), together with (3) *marked disorientation* and (4) *suggestibility*.

(b) *Alzheimer's Disease* is regarded by most authorities as synonymous with Presbyophrenia and only described separately because of the addition of *focal signs*, reflected in speech disorders and impairment of perception. There is *Aphasia* (failure to understand or reproduce speech), *Paraphasia* (distorted speech—'jargon'), *Agnosia* (failure to interpret correctly sense impressions) and *Apraxia* (failure to use objects correctly).

(c) *Pick's Disease*, occurring twice as frequently in women as in men, is of rare occurrence and is associated with circumscribed atrophy of the cortex and generally with a familiar history. Its symptomatology does not unduly differ from Alzheimer's Disease.

*Group* 5       *Involutional Melancholia*

Involutional Psychoses, which include those mental diseases occurring in association with the involutional period of life (in women between 40 and 50 years of age and between 55 to 65 years of age in men). The chief psychosis occurring at this period is described as (1) *Involutional Melancholia*, though other authorities describe (2) *a Paranoid type*.

(1) *Involutional Melancholia* exhibits the main characteristics of the depressive phase of the Manic-Depressive Psychosis, but anxiety and apprehension are more marked and the delusions tend to be either of a hypochondriacal or nihilistic type and generally centre round sin or death (the 'unpardonable sin').

(2) *A Paranoid type* of psychosis is also described during the involutional period. This is characterised by the more usual features of true Paranoia, with delusions of persecution, etc., but it is difficult to demonstrate any feature distinguishing it from Paranoia proper, even in prognosis.

*Group* 6       *The Epileptic Psychoses*

*The Epileptic Psychoses* (from the Greek, 'Epilepsia'—taking hold of, a seizure) cover a number of mental syndromes or states associated with the various forms of epilepsy and classified, in relation to the epileptic seizure, into (A) *Pre-Paroxysmal*, (B) *Inter-Paroxysmal*, (C) *Post-Paroxysmal* and (D) *Terminal*.

(A) *The Pre-Paroxysmal* state is, merely, an accentuation of the temperamental peculiarities associated with the epileptic constitution or character. This is reflected in sudden behaviour changes, consisting of general restlessness and irritability with a tendency to querulousness and aggressiveness, which precedes the prodromal or aura stage, signalling the onset of the convulsion.

(B) *The Inter-Paroxysmal* state refers to the epileptic character or constitution so prominent a characteristic of the epileptic psychotic. It is regarded by some authorities, notably the American Psychologist, Pierce Clark, as merely an intensification of the so-called epileptic make-up which is thought to exist in the pre-convulsive life of most epileptics. The chief features of the epileptic character constitute a quartet of symptoms, generally constant, comprising (1) *Simplicity*, (2) *Religiosity*, (3) *Irritability* and (4) *Querulousness*. Other features, such as selfishness, sexual excesses, resentment of disciplinary control, etc., may also be noted but they lack the constancy of the above four traits. These latter are readily recognised by the mental infantilism of the patient, the tendency to prayer and religious activities at most inappropriate times and places. The irritability of temperament is reflected in the inordinate display of temper on the most trivial provocation and there is a noticeable inclination to pick quarrels and to register complaints which are generally without foundation.

(C) *The Post-Paroxysmal* mental states are described as clouded states which either—follow convulsions, such as (1) *Automatism* and *Hystero-Epilepsy* or replace the convulsions and described as (2) *Epileptic Equivalents*.

(1) *Post-Epileptic Automatism*, generally following *Petit Mal*, consists of simple actions, some of an embarrassing nature, which are performed unconsciously with complete amnesia for the events subsequently. Hysterical convulsions,

following epileptic seizures, have also been described.

(2) *Epileptic Equivalents*, substituting convulsions, are of two types: (a) *Transient* and (b) *Prolonged*. The former, usually lasting from a few minutes to a few hours, consist generally of impulsive acts of violence known as *Epileptic Foror*, often leading to fatal results. *The Prolonged Equivalents*, lasting from some days to several months, may take the form of *Automatism* (double consciousness), as described above or may be exhibited in attacks of excitement, depression, confusion and even stupor (described as Epileptic Catatonia) as well as prolonged sleep (Narcolepsy).

(D) *The Terminal* or stage of deterioration (Epileptic Dementia) is exhibited in the chronic epileptic by the gradual deterioration of intellect, with poverty of ideation, emotional dulling and speech defect (plateau speech). Amnesia becomes more profound and the progressive nature of the disease leads to the 'wet and dirty stage.'

The occupational treatment of the epileptic, because of both the mental and physical disorder, calls for very special consideration. Epileptics must be graded according to mental and physical capacity. Crafts must also be graded to meet the individual needs as well as the general nature of the disease. The placement of the treatment must take into consideration the dangers involved in the sudden onset of the convulsive attacks and the selection of crafts will, likewise, be governed by the nature of the craft equipment and materials from the point of view of minimising risks of physical injury. Basketry and raffiacraft are eminently suitable in recommended cases as well as the very simple types of crafts in the case of deteriorated patients, such as rag-teasing and very light sanding.

## Group 7                    *The Alcoholic Psychoses*

*The Alcoholic Psychoses* cover a wide range of acute as well as chronic states, whose importance from the O.T. point of view may be gauged from the equally wide range of symptoms occurring in the various forms of mental disease associated with alcohol.

They may be listed schematically as follows:—

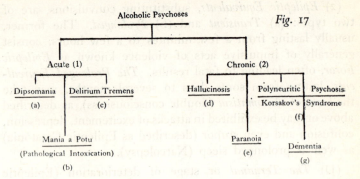

Fig. 17

1. The *Acute Alcoholic Psychoses* comprise three conditions, as listed, but cases of Mania à Potu and Delirium Tremens are rarely submitted for treatment in the public mental hospitals.

(A) *Dipsomania* is regarded by some authorities as merely a recurrent manic-depressive condition associated with alcoholic indulgence—the craving for alcohol being absent in the intervals between attacks. Undoubtedly the condition is recurrent but the extent and special feature of the alcoholic nature of the condition justify its special clinical recognition. There is often prodromal depression with irritability and insomnia before each attack and mental acuity tends to lessen after a number of attacks. The absence of alcoholic craving and indulgence in the intervals between attacks is a noteworthy feature.

(B) *Mania à Potu*, known also as *Pathological Intoxication*, is a state of frenzy or maniacal furor, occurring in susceptible individuals after ingestion of even very small quantities of alcohol and associated with marked confusion, hallucinations and illusions. The emotional changes are so profound that homicide or suicide may occur even during the very short duration of each attack, rarely more than 24 hours. There is complete amnesia for all incidents of each attack.

(C) *Delirium Tremens* is an acute condition occurring in a case of chronic alcoholism, arising either from marked continuous over-indulgence or more often from sudden abstinence following a prolonged bout of drinking. An attack may be precipitated in a chronic alcoholic, following an injury or an acute illness.

The condition is really an acute toxic confusional psychosis, accompanied by hallucinations of a terrifying type. In addition, there is marked restlessness, anxiety and apprehension with distractibility of attention. Conduct becomes very disordered, due to the delusions and hallucinations present, with subsequent amnesia for all events of the attack. Physically, the usual signs of chronic alcoholism are present— tremors, constipation, anorexia, fast pulse, etc.

2. *Chronic Alcoholism* covers a number of conditions, as listed, showing marked variations in symptomatology. Alcohol, like syphilis, may produce pathological changes in many different organs and parts of the body. Even in the brain, variations are likewise prominent. For this reason, the mental picture in chronic alcoholism shows many variations. Where hallucinations predominate, we describe the conditions as (d) *Alcoholic Hallucinosis*. With persecutory delusions crowding the picture, we get (e) *Alcoholic Paranoia*.

(F) *Polyneuritic Psychosis* (*Korsakov's Syndrome*) is a special mental condition appearing in cases of chronic alcoholism associated with Polyneuritis and other physical signs of the latter disease. The mental syndrome is reflected in the special disorders of memory present. There is amnesia of both the anterograde (recent) and retrograde (remote) type, as well as *paramnesia* (distorted memory) which consists of pseudo-reminiscences or falsifications of the memory, leading to what is described as *confabulation*. The memory, failing to function normally, because of errors in recognition, compensates by describing imaginary past 'experiences' that never occurred. There are also present hallucinations and well marked imperception with disorientation. The emotional tone is elated and euphoric, with grandiose ideas.

(G) *Alcoholic Dementia* is the terminal mental condition, seen in chronic alcoholism, following the continuous ingestion of alcohol over a very prolonged period of time. There is both intellectual and moral deterioration, the extent of which is determined by the amount of degeneration present in the brain substance, coverings and blood vessels, similar to those found in Senile Dementia. The mental symptoms may show some resemblance to the presenile psychoses by the presence of amnesia and paramnesia with complete disorientation. The persistence of hallucinations, however, in the condition is a factor of importance in differential diagnosis.

*Group* 8           *Syphilitic Psychoses*

Syphilitic Psychoses may be classified broadly into three types: (A) *Encephalitic* (Dementia Paralytica), (B) *Cerebral* (Meningeal and Vascular), and (C) *Tabetic* (Tabo-Paresis).

(A) *The Encephalitic* or *Parenchymatous* type, is also known as *General Paralysis of the Insane, General Paresis* or *Dementia Paralytica*. This psychosis occurs, generally from two to twenty years after primary infection with syphilis, although the percentage of infects developing the psychosis is as low as two. The mental symptoms are usually described in three stages—(1) *The initial* or *prodromal stage*, (2) *The Paretic* or *fully developed stage* and (3) *The Terminal* or *final stage.*

(1) *The prodromal* or early symptoms, which develop insidiously, consist of gradual personality changes with general intellectual and moral deterioration. Normal inhibitions are lost, leading to alcoholic and sexual excesses, with neglect of personal cleanliness and tidiness. Judgment becomes impaired with development of delusions, which tend to be grandiose. Defect of memory occurs, with marked forgetfulness regarding appointments. Physical signs are also present, consisting mainly of (a) *slurring of speech,* (b) *facial or other tremors* (thrombone movement of the tongue), (c) *exaggeration of knee reflexes* (not constant) and (d) *Argyll-Robertson pupil* (reacting to accommodation, but not to light).

(2) *The Paretic Stage* is so called because of the development of convulsions, but these may, in some cases, appear in the early stage of the disease. In the fully developed stage, all the prodromal features show accentuation. Disorders of memory become more profound with marked intellectual

impairment and disorientation. The physical signs also become more pronounced with the development of apoplectiform attacks of various types (with speedy recovery from each attack). Muscular weakness is also noticeable, but there is a rather marked increase in weight. The general picture has been described as 'fat, fatuous and fitty,' leading ultimately, in the absence of early treatment, to the (3) *Terminal Stage*, where the patient becomes bedridden, wet and dirty, leading a purely vegetative existence, with further increase in the general mental and physical deterioration.

A number of varieties of the disease have been described according to the prominence of any special symptom, such as (a) *convulsive*, (b) *depressive*, (c) *maniacal*, (d) *circular* (manic-depressive type), (e) *stuporose*, (f) *demented* and (g) *expansive* (delusions of grandeur prominent). These clinical divisions are of importance from the O.T. point of view as they indicate the main mental state present, which will influence the type of craft treatment to be prescribed.

(B) *Cerebral* or *Interstitial Syphilis*, affecting mainly the meninges and blood vessels, gives rise to mental symptoms of a varying character, dependent on the site and extent of the interstitial involvement. These mental symptoms, accordingly, may range from excitement to depression and even delirium and confusion. They may occasionally be represented by a dull, pseudo-stuporose state, with loss of sphincter control. Hallucinations and delusions may also be present, with such memory defects as amnesia and paramnesia (confabulation). There may also be associated physical symptoms and signs, chiefly headache (nocturnal), insomnia with vertigo and often vomiting. The physical signs mainly in evidence are cranial nerve involvement (all cranial nerves may be attacked—generally the third). Optic neuritis and atrophy may also appear and convulsive and epileptiform seizures, including apoplectiform attacks, are not uncommon.

(C) *Tabo-Paresis* may be preceded or followed by mental symptoms, also of a variable content. These may include phases of the manic-depressive psychosis, even the circular types, as well as confusion and anxiety, complicated by hallucinations. Kraepelin expressed the opinion that the most common mental symptom associated with Tabes Dorsalis is an acute hallucinatory form of excitement.

*Group* 9                              *The Psychoneuroses*

*The Psychoneuroses* constitute a benign type of mental disorder, represented by psychological conflict which usually gives rise to subjective symptoms or may be expressed in outward physical manifestations, for which there is no organic basis. These symptoms, the nature of which is not appreciated by the patient, subserve a special purpose in his mental life, without leading to anti-social behaviour. The symptoms may represent a disguised form of gratification of subconscious strivings and desires or may act as a protection against these repressed desires by a process of substitution.

*The Psychoneuroses* were formerly distinguished from conditions classified as *Neuroses* on the plea that the associated mental and bodily symptoms of the latter were governed mainly, if not entirely, by physical factors. The modern tendency is to discard the latter designation on the grounds that, in all such conditions, the psychological elements, even when disguised, constitute the important factor in the psychosomatic symptom-content. Accordingly, such disorders as neurasthenia and hysteria fall readily under the definition of the Psychoneuroses given above. On the other hand, the psychoses proper cover a wide range of disorders, where the psychological elements dominate the symptomatology, irrespective of the presence or extent of somatic changes. Nevertheless, it is difficult to draw any definite line of demarcation between the two, but recognised points of difference may be tabulated as on opposite page.

There is no uniform classification of the Psychoneuroses, though that of Freud or some modification of it, is the most universally accepted, recognising four main forms:—

1. *Neurasthenia,* 2. *Compulsive States* (Psychasthenia), 3. *Hysteria* and 4. *Anxiety States.*

1. *Neurasthenia,* first distinguished by Beard in 1868, is described as a state of simple nervous exhaustion, associated

| POINTS | PSYCHOSES | PSYCHONEUROSES |
|---|---|---|
| 1. Personality | Markedly Disorganised. (Total Reaction of Meyer). | Very Slightly Disorganised. (Partial Reaction of Meyer). |
| 2. Disorders of Judgment. (Delusions) | Very Common | Absent—though there may be over-valuation of ideas. |
| 3. Reality Interpretation | Greatly Disturbed | Unchanged. |
| 4. Conation | Behaviour greatly disturbed. | Only very slightly disordered. |
| 5. Emotional Disturbances | Very Frequent | Not Pronounced. |
| 6. Herd Instinct | Uusally lost | Generally retained. |
| 7. Insight | Usually illness not recognised as such. | Conscious wish to get well, though subconscious desires may be to the contrary. |

with general mental and physical fatigue, including diminished power of concentration with irritability and insomnia. Several different varieties are described according to the predominant nature of the symptoms present, particularly in regard to localisation, such as (a) Cardiac and Circulatory Forms, (b) Gastric Form, (c) Cerebral and Spinal, (d) Sensory and (e) Genital types.

2. *Psychasthenia* (*Foliè de Doute*) is the term used by Janet for the various obsessional and anxiety states, distinguishing them from Hysteria. It is now generally confined to the psychoneurotic conditions, which exhibit obsessions, whether of a phobiacal, compulsive or impulsive nature. The obsessional state may arise in the (a) *emotional,* (b) *volitional* or (c) *intellectual fields.* (a) *Emotional obsessions* are represented by various phobias, such as Claustrophobia (fear of being in a closed space), Monophobia (fear of being alone), etc. (b) *Volitional obsessions* are seen in the various manias or compulsions, such as Kleptomania (compulsive tendency to

steal), Pyromania (tendency to set fire to objects), etc.

(c) *Intellectual obsessions* occur as doubts and indecisions, such as failure to decide on or accept one of two courses of action. As examples of these may be cited the doubts that arise in regard to the performance of certain actions, such as posting a letter or locking a particular door before retiring at night, and the state of indecision that may arise as to which shoe to put on first, etc.

3. *Hysteria* has been described as the production of abnormalities in various mental and bodily functions, as a result of psychological conflict, without any organic basis or cause for such mal-functioning. It is accordingly a purposeful, though unconscious type of mental reaction, which produces a train of symptoms, acting as a disguise, in substitution for the fulfilment of a desire, which cannot be consciously gratified. These substitutive symptoms, having no organic basis, are merely assumed and consequently most organic diseases may be simulated in hysteria, such as paralysis (all types), disturbances of sensation, including vision and hearing and other physical ailments. Even mental disturbances may be simulated, such as amnesias, fugues (changing to a new occupation and mode of life with subsequent complete amnesia for all events occurring during the fugue), somnambulism and trance states, as well as stupor, confusional and maniacal phases.

Different types of Hysteria have been distinguished. Janet described (a) *Conversion Hysteria* and (b) *Anxiety Hysteria*, but the latter is now included among the Anxiety States. *Fixation Hysteria* is also differentiated, but this is merely a special type of Conversion Hysteria, where the physical arrangement is fixed in one special part of the body, such as one limb.

4. *Anxiety States* represent a form of mental disturbance, which may occur in association with many bodily illnesses, psychoses and other psychoneuroses, constituting a prominent and important symptom in any of these latter, or it may occur as a psychoneurosis *sui generis*, where the anxiety appears as the primary symptom. The latter *Anxiety State*

proper may be described as a condition of apprehension, with the emotional reaction of fear and resulting in a number of disquieting bodily symptoms, which tend to create a feeling of impending disaster. The bodily symptoms are as varied as they are numerous and are generally of a hypochondriacal nature. They consist mainly of cardiac, respiratory and digestive disturbances as well as insomnia, terrifying dreams, vertigo, etc.

*The Occupational Treatment of the Psychoneuroses* cannot be prescribed on any system of general principles that are universally applicable. Psychoneurotic conditions exhibit such a varied symptomatology, covering such a wide field, that each case must be dealt with as a separate and individual problem. Two factors, however, demand prior attention—(1) the nature of the associated physical symptoms and (2) the prevailing mental state.

(1) The former must receive primary consideration, as the physical condition will determine whether O.T. is desirable, particularly in the acute stages, as for instance in neurasthenia; and if O.T. is not contraindicated, a decision must be reached as to the suitability of recreational as against handicraft treatment. Broadly, recreational therapy, particularly the development of an attractive hobby, may be more serviceable in the psychoneuroses, owing to its strongly externalising influence in combating the deep-seated introversion, so prominent in the latter. Psychoneurotics are excessively wrapt up in themselves and in their psychological and physical problems and there is nothing equal to recreational treatment, particularly the active, non-passive type, to promote extroversion. Such treatment, however, must be in close association with any psychotherapeutic procedure adopted. A judicious blending of psychotherapy and recreational therapy constitutes the strongest and most successful method of dealing with the difficult and often intractable problem of treatment of the psychoneurotic. Craft therapy may not be ruled out in certain isolated cases, where the physical state presents no barrier and where handicraft, rather than a recreational project, may make greater appeal.

(2) Whether recreational or craft measures are adopted, the prevailing mental state will influence the type of O.T. to be prescribed. Depression will call for stimulative types of crafts or recreations, while agitation and anxiety will require more sedative measures.

# CHAPTER XII.

## PSYCHOLOGICAL ANALYSIS *(contd.)*

### Mental States

(B) Mental States, as distinct from individual mental diseases refer to the prevailing symptom-content in the psychotic, as represented by the current emotional tone, with the associated intellectual and behaviour disorders. Such states as *Excitement* (with or without elation), *Depression, Anxiety, Confusion, Stupor, Apathy, Delirium,* etc., irrespective of the causative mental disease in each case, require separate study and analysis for occupational therapy purposes. The recognition of these states and their due appraisal in regard to craft application is of much greater importance for the occupational therapy personnel than the detailed evaluation of the psychoses which gives rise to these states. The same type of mental disease is rarely represented by identical features in any two persons. Such factors as personality, character, temperament, environmental influences, etc., will tend to create individual deviations from the standard and accepted representation of the disease. For this reason, *occupational therapy must be correlated more with the predominating mental state than with the original psychosis.* In other words, the symptoms are submitted for treatment rather than the disease itself and hence craft analysis must be governed primarily by this principle.

### 1—*Excitement*

(1) *Increased Psychomotor Activity,* referred to generally as *Excitement,* is a well-recognised mental state occurring in a number of psychoses. It is seen in its most typical form in (A) *Mania,* but even in the latter, it may vary in intensity from the mild restlessness of hypomania to the

extreme continuous press of activity, both physical and mental, in the fully-developed stage of acute mania. The excitement of mania, therefore, while of varying intensity, is specially characterised both in its accompanying elation and particularly by its prolonged, continuous nature. It is these special features which distinguish it from similar states occurring in other psychoses. (B) In *Schizophrenia*, the type of restlessness and excitement, as seen in the active stage of katatonia, is of the impulsive and intermittent type. It also varies in intensity from mild agitation to extreme turbulence, but is generally of short duration—from a few hours to a few days and the element of elation is lacking. (C) In the *Senile Psychoses*, a degree of restlessness and excitement is seen in the form described as Senile Mania, as well as in the 'occupational delirium of the presenile psychoses.' These take the form more of increased irritability with associated insomnia and are complicated by both memory and intellectual failure. Simple, sedative occupations will create a suitable outlet for the purposeless activity of the senile dement, as well as counteracting the associated insomnia. (D) In the *Epileptic Psychoses*, there is mild agitation in both the pre-convulsive and post-convulsive periods, which is generally an exacerbation of the epileptic temperament, as already described and generally of short duration. *The Epileptic Equivalent* known as *Epileptic Furor*, whether transient or prolonged, is an extreme form of excitement, characterised by its impulsive and highly dangerous nature. In both cases, occupational treatment is not indicated and active precautionary measures have to be substituted. (E) Motor excitement shows many variations in intensity in the *Alcoholic Psychoses*, ranging from mild irritability and agitation in Dipsomania to the more extreme restlessness of Delirium Tremens and the maniacal frenzy of Mania à Potu (Pathological Intoxication). The latter, owing to its sudden nature and generally brief duration, has no O.T. significance and only in the convalescent stage of Delirium Tremens may occupational therapy be successfully pressed into use. As an adjunct in the general prophylactic attack on alcoholism, particularly in the early stages, craft and

recreational treatment can play a most important role.
(F) *The Syphilitic Psychoses*, particularly the manic variety
of these conditions, show a certain amount of restlessness
and excitement of varying intensity. Active malarial treatment
is of primary importance here and is usefully supplemented
by O.T. in the convalescent stage. (G) Maniacal phases or
states of excitement occur with varying intensity in other
*psychoses*, such as those *associated with drug addiction, infectious diseases, circulatory disturbances*, etc. In each of these
types of cases, where suitable, a sedative occupation may be
prescribed appropriate to the intensity and nature of the
excitement present.

## 2—*Depression*

(2) *States of Depression* are of relative importance in
frequency and require very careful analysis for O.T. prescription and application. As with the restlessness in Mania,
they present marked variations in intensity and are seen in
their most typical form in (1) *Melancholia. Depression* may
be described in general terms as the converse of Mania.
Here the hyper-functioning of all parts of the body, reflected
in the general excitement occurring in the latter, is
replaced by marked retardation of all activities, even to the
extent of manifest flexion of the extremities including the
arms and a general state of inertia, as already described.
The prevailing state of depression may be complicated and
even entirely governed by co-existing delusions.

Stimulative occupations are indicated in depressive states,
but due cognisance must be given to (1) the *concomitant
physical disturbances* as well as (2) the *associated suicidal
tendency*. (1) The physical changes, as evidenced by the
flexion and restriction of joint movements, so pronounced
in the early acute stages, rather limit the range of stimulating
crafts available. Recourse must be had to the very simplest
of the minor crafts at first, which, while of the stimulative
type, must embrace only movements of very restricted
amplitude, but of such a nature as to arouse the patient's
interests. With the gradual development of muscular relaxation and consequent increased competency in performance,

there should be an accompanying, though gradual increase in the element of complexity, in passing from the simpler to the less simple crafts.

(2) The use of crafts for depressed cases must never ignore the possibility of suicidal impulse and this will further limit the range of suitable occupations. Crafts that might induce or facilitate the accomplishment of suicidal ideas, either by the type of tools in use or the nature of the materials required, are strictly contraindicated, even in the convalescing stages of Depression. Consequently, two points of importance demanding recognition stand out in this respect, (A) *Every melancholic is a potential suicide* and (B) *the milder the depression, the greater the tendency towards suicide,* and this is unfortunately true of the convalescing melancholic, even when approaching the point of recovery.

States of depression, apart from the most typical forms seen in the various types of melancholia, occur also as a prominent symptom in the course of many other psychoses. In these latter, however, they are of a more transient nature, but, as long as they tend to dominate the symptom-content, they call for the recognition and detail in treatment outlined above, due regard being paid to the other allied and often equally important symptoms occurring in these psychoses.

2. *Senile Melancholia* represents a depressive phase, that may obtrude itself upon the course of the degenerative processes occurring in senile dementia. The depression here has the general characteristics already described, but is complicated by the presence of the various other features of the disease. The failure of concentrated attention, as well as the prevailing irritability, agitation and disturbance of recent memory create an O.T. problem that is peculiar to old age. The marked diminution in the physical activities of the senile patient is an additional complication. All these call for a type of occupation that is both stimulative and sedative; stimulative to counteract the depression and sedative to check the agitation and mild restlessness. Such a therapeutic 'vicious circle', however, cannot be reduced to a common denominator, applicable to all such cases. Each individual case must be considered on its merits. One must

decide whether craft or recreational treatment forms the best recommendation. The nature of the predominant symptoms in any particular case will influence a decision in this respect and will help to indicate the type of craft or recreation best suited for treatment.

3. The depression occurring in *Involutional Melancholia* does not differ in general features from that of the manic-depressive Psychosis. The element of anxiety, however, is more pronounced and because of the possible tendency towards suicide, emphasis must be placed on the precautions already outlined.

4. A depressive phase may also be seen in *Dementia Paralytica* (G.P.I.), in which delusions of a nihilistic type are present, as well as suicidal impulses, but these are mainly transient features in the course of the disease. Their recognition in appropriate craft prescription is called for, as long as they cloud the general symptomatological picture.

5. Depression may constitute the main feature of many other psychoses, such as those associated with Paralysis Agitans, Huntingdon's Chorea and various bodily diseases and infections, including Epidemic Encephalitis (Encephalitis Lethargica), etc. The depressive phase occurring in all these diseases does not exhibit any special features that are not common to all melancholic states and does not create any additional problem in occupational treatment, apart from any special physical difficulties that may be present.

### 3—Anxiety

3. *Anxiety* is a well-recognised mental state, that may occur in association with or independent of depression. In the latter case it is seen most typically in the *Psychoneurotic Anxiety State. Anxiety* may be described as a state of mental distress varying in intensity from that of mild concern to extreme apprehension arising from the continuous contemplation of unpleasant possibilities and associated with an emotional reaction of fear. It is a natural and healthy reaction to exercise concern for situations that may lead to dangerous or undesirable results and this helps to make suitable provision in dealing with such difficulties. When the concern, however, develops

into a state of prolonged anxiety, confining itself to a morbid subjective foreboding, without adequate adjustment to the situation, the condition becomes abnormal. Anxiety may, thus, vary in degree from that of the normal, healthy reaction as described, through its various psychoneurotic manifestations, to its most extreme form, when it becomes linked to a full-fledged melancholic psychosis.

Anxiety may occur as an auxiliary symptom in many psychoses, but, in the psychoneurotic anxiety state proper, it is the main, predominating symptom. Associated with the condition of anxiety is a state of chronic tension with general irritability and extreme self-centring and the numerous bodily symptoms arising from the accompanying emotional reaction of fear. The occupational treatment must, therefore, be organised on the lines laid down for the psychoneuroses in general, as already described. Where craft procedures are unsuitable, because of the physical concomitants of the anxiety condition, recreational therapy will play a very important role. But here, also, passive amusement will have to replace active physical exercise in individual cases. Recreations of the active type, however, particularly the acquisition of an interesting and attractive hobby, when this is not contraindicated, will produce the best results. The ability to achieve something worth while, even under the guise of a simple hobby, will tend to promote self-reliance and a healthy adjustment towards the mental conflict and tension associated with the anxiety state. Occupational treatment on these lines, linked with appropriate psychotherapy, will forge the only satisfactory weapon in attacking this psychoneurotic disorder.

### 4—Confusion (Delirium and Stupor)

Confusion may be described as a state of disorientation (inability to locate oneself in time or place) following clouding of consciousness arising from the effects of toxins, exhaustion or dementia. Toxins circulating in the body, whether arising from acute infections, drugs, the puerperium, etc., tend to cause a clouding of consciousness, leading to a confusional state. The latter will vary in depth from a very mild form through various stages of delirium to its most profound form, including stupor. In the non-delirious and non-stuporose form of confusion, the clouding of consciousness is not sufficiently deep to eliminate reponses to sensory stimuli. The latter are merely subject to misinterpretation with consequent imperception, leading to disorientation, with mild purposeless motor restlessness. In *Delirium,* the dimming of consciousness may vary in extent from mild delirium to its most extreme form of acute delirious mania, but is characterised by the usual features of confusion as above, and, in addition, there are typical hallucinations, with restlessness and noisy incoherency.

In *True Stupor* there is definite clouding of consciousness, referred to as 'dissociation of consciousness,' with failure to comprehend sensory impressions and with all voluntary activity in abeyance. There is complete indifference to environment and even personal needs, necessitating tube feeding. The most extreme form has been described as *Anergic Stupor.* As stated already, what is described as 'Katatonic Stupor' is not a true stupor, as the state of inertia and apathy present is incorrectly interpreted as a clouding of consciousness; whereas sensory impressions are registering quite normally.

Confusional phases have been noted in the course of other psychoses, but they are generally associated with some toxic element present and are usually of a transitory nature.

The *occupational treatment* of confusional states depends largely on the general mental and physical condition and the degree of confusion present. In the acute stages, where imperception and disorientation are most pronounced, as well as in the extreme cases of delirium and stupor, both the mental and physical condition will be a definite contra-indication for O.T. It is in the convalescent stages of the disorder that O.T. will give the best results and whether it will be on craft or recreational lines, or both, will depend on each case individually. The medical prescription will be governed by the requirements in each instance, where the mental and physical factors will have been subjected to careful and exhaustive analysis so as to arrive at the most appropriate form of treatment.

## 5—Mental Apathy

5. *Mental Apathy* is a disorder in the affective sphere and has been described as emotional indifference. Emotional disorders may occur either as (A) *Affective Dulling* or *Affective Loss* (Athymia) or (B) *Emotional Dysharmony* or *Emotional Displacement* (Parathymia), already referred to as distortion of emotion. Mental apathy or affective dulling is a positive loss of normal emotional functioning. It is characterised by a complete emotional indifference to pleasurable or painful situations. Experiences, that normally elicit emotional responses of pleasure or pain, fail to produce such reactions in cases exhibiting emotional dulling or mental apathy. Such cases may remain completely unmoved in the presence of the most heartrending situations. The news of the death of a very near relative may be received with a most inappropriate air of unconcern and in such as those suffering from Schizophrenia, this emotional dulling may be complicated by emotional displacement (Dysharmony) represented by silly giggling or alternate weeping.

There is a notable tendency to confuse this state of mental apathy with that of depression as already referred to in describing Katatonia. The mental apathy arises from the poverty of emotion and thus explains the absence of any subjective feeling, such as that of sadness or the feeling of unhappiness, which characterises depression. It is, accordingly, referred to as pseudo-depression. Emotional dulling or apathy is most frequently encountered in Schizophrenia, particularly in the hebephrenic and katatonic forms. It is also seen in the presenile Dementias, as well as Senile Dementia Paralytica (G.P.I.). In these latter conditions, emotional deterioration may be very profound, dependent on the extent of organic changes present. The emotional, as well as the intellectual changes, occurring in these Dementia Psychoses will place occupational procedures on a purely symptomatic basis, on the general lines already laid down.

In cases of Schizophrenia, however, the mental indifference

is mainly a reflexion of the state of introversion, evidenced by the retreat from reality and objective happenings. This withdrawal of interest from the external environment to a world of self-created phantasy, represents the most extreme form of introversion. It is this lack of interest in externals that creates the appearance of emotional dulling. This apparent affective disorder arises from this withdrawal of interest rather than to any positive emotional disorder *per se*. The attention to phantasy and the disregard for reality so prominent a feature of the introversion of the Schizophrenic has been described as a regression to infantile or primitive levels. It is in cases of this extreme type of emotional dulling and general apathy that occupational treatment is directed on re-educational lines. *Re-educational Therapy*, which, as already described, is a special combination of handicraft and recreational procedures in a 24-hour balanced programme of work, rest and play, constituting a very successful method of Habit-Training. Where mental apathy is seen in its most profound form, as in the regressed Schizophrenic, Re-educational Therapy is the method of choice. It represents the simplest of craft and recreational procedures and its success in the habit-training of 'wet and dirty' cases, as already detailed, may be satisfactorily extended to other types of schizoid regression, even to those characterised mainly by emotional dulling and general mental apathy. The resuscitation of former habits of work and activity as well as the creation of new habits and interests, so successfully achieved by re-educational methods, may prove the only means of countering this condition of schizoid introversion.

### Mental Types or Temperaments (Personality)

*Personality* may be described as the mental and physical make-up which conditions each individual's reactions and responses to different situations. No two persons may react in a completely identical manner in the same set of circumstances. It has been defined by Katz as 'the behaviour of the individual which differentiates him from his fellows.' McDougall states that 'disposition, temper and temperament are the raw materials of personality provided by heredity.'

*Temperament* is difficult to define clearly and simply. It may be described as the prevailing mental attitude and life mood of the individual as governed mainly by the general biochemical activities of his organism. Some people have a bright and cheerful temperament, while others tend to be morose and gloomy. McDougall has written that:—

> 'The temperament of a man may be provisionally defined as the sum of the effects upon his mental life of the metabolic or chemical changes that are constantly going on in all the tissues of his body.'

It is a well-recognised fact that the ingestion of alcohol, even in moderate quantities, tends to alter temperament. Alcohol has been noted to transform the shy, retiring and timid person into a most aggressive, buoyant and self-assertive individual.

Many workers have essayed a classification of individuals based on physique and mental traits. Even in olden times, the Hindus recognised three symbolical types, namely, the Bull, the Horse and the Hare. The famous German professor, Kretschmer, differentiated four bodily types, each associated with special mental characteristics, as follows: (1) *The Asthenic Type*, (2) *The Pyknic Type*, (3) *The Athletic Type* and (4) *The Dyplastic Type*.

1. *The Asthenic Type* is represented by the tall, lean and bony class of individual, with stooped and narrow shoulders and flattened chest. In temperament, this type is of the retiring, introverted and sensitive, shy type, classified as schizothymic (Bleuler's Schizoid).

2. *The Pyknic Type* is characterised by the short, stocky and fat figure, with rounded chest and head. Temperamentally, this type shows variations in mood from cheerfulness to sadness and referred to as cyclothymic (Bleuler's syntonic).

3. *The Athletic Type* is the muscular, broad-shouldered, well-built individual and represented as being midway between the pyknic and asthenic types. The temperament in this type tends more to the Schizoid than Cycloid.

4. *The Dyplastic* represents a mixed type in physique and is characterised by various glandular abnormalities,

giving rise to such conditions as myxoedma, infantilism or eunuchoidism, etc. The associated temperament is generally of the Schizoid type.

Analysis of these four types are only of O.T. importance in the differentiation and recognition of the two temperaments —(1) The Cyclothymic (Cycloid) and (2) the Schizothymic (Schizoid). The former is associated with the manic-depressive phychosis and the latter with Schizophrenia. Jung, distinguishing these two types as (1) Extroverts and (2) Introverts, respectively, wrote as follows:—

'The two types are so essentially different, presenting so striking a contrast, that their existence even to the uninitiated in psychological matters becomes an obvious fact, when once attention has been drawn to it. Who does not know those taciturn, impenetrable, often shy natures, who form such a vivid contrast to those other open, sociable, serene maybe, or at least friendly and accessible characters, who are on good terms with all the world, or even when disagreeing with it, still hold a relation to it, by which they and it are mutually affected?'

*Introversion*, as opposed to *Extroversion*, has already been referred to briefly, when dealing with Schizophrenia. Each constitutes the mental attitude, in its adjustment to life's problems, as exhibited by the manner in which the individual's interests are directed, whether self-centred, denoting *Introversion* or concerned more with external reality as in *Extroversion*. These characteristics of temperament described by Jung and applicable to normals are readily distinguishable in psychotic cases. The acute maniac, in his general psychomotor activity, is more preoccupied with objects and activities in his immediate environment than with ideas of personal interest. On the other hand, the Schizophrenic withdraws from reality and becomes absorbed in his own dream world, exhibiting introversion in its most extreme form.

While the occupational treatment of these two mental types will be influenced, to a large extent, by the associated psychotic disturbance present, special recognition must be given to any element of *introversion* in the symptomatology.

Occupational therapy possesses a special property in breaking through the barrier of mental inaccessibility set up by introversion and restoring the patient's normal interests in the daily activities external to him. Stimulative occupations tend to rouse the patient's interests objectively and renew his former healthy contacts with his environment. They help to transfer attention from the self-created world of phantasy to the external world of reality, by encouraging normal emotional reactions.

*Extroversion*, which represents an exaggerated and over-interest in the immediate environment to the exclusion of personal interests and requirements, calls for the sedative type of occupation. This type of O.T. tends to restore the normal balance between self and reality, between subjective and objective interests and exercises a restraining influence on overactivity, as seen in most psychotic extroverts. The most extreme form of extroversion, as seen in the acute maniac, is complicated by the associated factors of 'flow of ideas' and distractibility of attention. The occupational prescription will be mostly concerned in recommending a craft that will tend to arouse interest and compel attention and possess an essentially sedative quality. This can only be satisfactorily determined by individual analysis—treating each case as a separate problem, which cannot be dealt with under any preconceived system of special principles.

# CHAPTER XIII.

## CRAFT ANALYSIS

### GENERAL

THE QUESTION of the selection of crafts suitable for occupational therapy purposes is one that immediately suggests itself in the very earliest stages of organisation. A detailed analysis and subsequent classification of suitable crafts will tend to simplify the problem of organisation, as well as facilitate the development and extension of the treatment in all its various phases. Several factors, mostly inter-related, require to be considered in dealing with this important question. The selection of crafts must be based on considerations of (1) *Therapeusis*, (2) *Complexity*, (3) *Adaptability*, (4) *Utility* and (5) *Quality*. (1) *Therapeusis*—Each craft is assessed, primarily, for its curative properties, which render this element of therapeusis a *sine qua non* condition of selection. From this it must be deduced that occupations, which have no treatment value, are automatically contraindicated. In this respect, however, it must be borne in mind that the curative value of a craft may be dependent on several co-existing factors—(a) *the type of patient under treatment*, (b) *the duration of treatment* and (c) *the complexity or otherwise of the craft.*

(a) *The mental and physical condition* of the patient will have an immediate bearing on the selection of a suitable occupation. This has been dealt with in detail in the psychological analysis of the patients requiring treatment. A craft which produces definite therapeutic results in a convalescing manic-depressive, may have a very injurious effect, if applied in the earlier stages of this disease. This apparently anomalous position is based on inter-related conditions, namely the complexity of the craft and the receptivity and operative ability of the patient. The fulfilment of an advanced and rather complicated task may be entirely dependent on a

191

certain alertness and keenness of mind that a fully developed
case of melancholia would not possess, particularly in the
early acute stage of the disease. Such a craft application
would prove not only non-therapeutic but distinctly harmful.
Contrariwise, the simple kindergarten type of craft, availed
of in the early stages of a mental disease, would have little
therapeutic value for the mental convalescent, mainly because
of its simplicity and monotonous, non-satisfying qualities.
This develops the important principle that *Craft-therapy
is regulated by the complexity of the craft in relation to the
mental state under treatment—the most important factor being
the type of patient submitted for treatment.*

(b) *The duration of treatment* also affects the therapeutic
value of a craft and must be adjusted to meet the individual
needs of patients. As already stated, the acute and early
stages of mental disease will affect the receptivity of a patient
and will thus restrict the therapeutic value of the treatment.
This is particularly so in connection with the mode and
duration of treatment. In the initial and early stages, periods
of treatment must be much shorter than usual with more
prolonged periods of rest and relaxation. The latter will
subsequently be reduced and the former increased, proportionately to the mental improvement attained. This leads
to the formulation of another important principle of craft
analysis, namely *that the work undertaken will be prescribed
in doses to suit the mental condition at the time of treatment.*
It follows, therefore, that overdosage may be as injurious
as underdosage may be ineffectual and, consequently, the
therapeutic quality of a task or craft will be dependent on
its applicability in terms of dosage. In other words, its
therapeutic effect will be influenced by the duration and mode
of operation.

(c) (2) *The complexity of crafts* has an important bearing
on their therapeutic assessment and their consequent suitability for selection. All crafts may be divided broadly into
*Simple* or *Complex*, based on their simplicity and ease of
operation or otherwise, but such a classification has only a
relative basis, due to its dependency on such factors as the
competency of the patient as well as the mental state pre-

vailing at the time of treatment. What might be simple for one patient might be difficult or complex for another patient, dependent on the past experiences of each, as well as factors of natural aptitude, interest, attraction, etc. Further, the mental condition would vary the simplicity or complexity of a craft by its effect on the patient's competency at the time of treatment.

Notwithstanding the manner in which the mental state at the time of treatment may vary the complexity value of crafts, a broad grading of occupations for general purposes into (1) *Simple*, (2) *Minor Complex* and (3) *Major Complex*, as with recreations, is essential to facilitate organisation, development and subsequent application. Every therapeutic craft will, therefore, be classified in one of these three divisions, apart from such factors as (3) *Adaptability*, (4) *Utility* and (5) *Quality*. This general division of the crafts will correspond broadly with the general classification of all mental cases into the three groups referred to in the Re-educational Therapy Section. The simpler crafts would be selected for Group I class of patients, while crafts of the lesser complex type would be available for Group II patients and major complex crafts for Group III, just as in the case of recreations.

It follows from this that many crafts may be so extremely complex from both the subjective viewpoint in the matter of comprehension of highly-involved techniques as well as objectively in the difficulty and intricacy of movement and performance, as to render them devoid of any element of therapeusis for most patients and consequently unsuitable, generally, for occupational therapy purposes. The assembling of delicate instruments and machines, where technical training and previous experience are essential, may be cited as examples. This raises another important question in craft selection, namely, *adaptability*.

(3) *Adaptability*. Many crafts may prove unsuitable for occupational therapy departments because of (a) extreme technical complexity, as those just referred to or (b) owing to the cumbersome and unwieldy nature of the necessary apparatus or materials. Considerations of space and the

absence of the element of finality in the processes of completion, would rule out the use of many crafts. Simplicity and portability of equipment are important considerations in influencing choice of selections. A craft involving several different processes of operation, each requiring bulky and extensive equipment, would be unsuitable for many reasons, not the least of which might prove the absence of adequate housing space as well as considerations of cost. Such factors as the bulky nature of the raw materials, as well as the possible multiple nature of the latter for any individual occupation, might render it unsuitable for similar reasons. In addition, a craft involving several different processes of operation, each with its own patient quota in control, would lack the element of individuality associated with the full completion of an article. The satisfaction and consequent therapeutic advantage derived in the initiation and final construction of a particular product by a patient or group of patients, must not be lost sight of in the selection of suitable crafts.

The element of adaptability is also a feature of many handicrafts, which renders them capable of adjustment to the various types of cases submitted for treatment. Weaving, basketry, etc., are important crafts, which are very highly adaptable for therapeutic purposes, by the ease in adjustment of working processes, from the very simple types, through the various grades of complexity to the very highly skilled and complex activities, associated with the more advanced forms of these crafts. Simple weaving on card looms, with its repetitive, monotonous movements, may be replaced, as required, by table looms, with somewhat more advanced weave designs and these again by large hand and pedal looms, involving more complicated reed movements, with twill and check designs, requiring more skill, attention and control. This feature of adaptability is actually a special *quality* of these crafts and is referred to again further on, under the latter heading.

(4) *Utility*. The choice of crafts should be influenced, though not exclusively, by the element of utility. This would be based on routine hospital requirements, where the introduction of crafts and occupations would provide products

and articles for the hospital that might, otherwise, have to be purchased from external sources.

In all large mental hospitals and particularly in the public institutions, there are many departments and sections which form part of the routine activity of hospital life from their very inception. These sections tend to be operated in some mental hospitals for economic and utility reasons in the absence of any organised occupational therapy services. Such sections, uninfluenced by therapeutic considerations, were concerned often with output and supply and their patient content based on physical performance rather than on the individual patient's needs and wishes and with no therapeutic objective. Included among these and referred to already as *Technical and Utility Sections* are (1) *The various Tradeshops*, (2) *The Engineering Department*, (3) *Farm and Garden*, (4) *The Bakery*, (5) *The Offices and Stores*, (6) *The Dining-halls*, (7) *The Laundry*, (8) *The Kitchen*, etc. All these sections have an utility purpose in meeting hospital needs and requirements, but, under therapeutical guidance in the occupational therapy department, they can be successfully re-organised to augment, substantially, the treatment services of the latter.

It is surprising to what extent the occupational therapy percentage is raised in a hospital where these utility services are fully developed under the auspices of the handicraft therapy department. The variety of work involved in the different sections heightens interest and provides an element of versatility and attractiveness, which is such an essential feature of the thoroughly organised occupational therapy department. They have the further advantage of being under skilled control, where technical advice is immediately available, which is capable of being directed and moulded into therapeutic grooves by the occupational therapist. They help considerably to provide advanced treatment for the convalescent and Group III type of patients.

The utility sections mentioned above are nearly all standard in most large mental hospitals and provide an important nucleus for the technical sections of the occupational therapy department but they can be usefully supplemented by the development of auxiliary sections to meet the needs of the hospital in other essential requirements. For instance, a cementcraft section will provide many commodities that would, otherwise, have to be purchased from outside sources, such as concrete blocks and bricks, roof tiles, floor tiles, sewer pipes, fence posts, garden ornaments, etc. The variety of moulds and machinery, as well as the use of cement in various colours for both floor and roof tiles, etc., provide a series of occupations in the one section, exhibiting as much versatility and attractiveness as simplicity in handling.

The wide range of work involved is easily taught and proficiency is quickly achieved, without even previous skilled experience. The introduction of colour-craft in the manufacture of floor tiles in various shapes and sizes, as well as roof and ridge tiles, renders the work attractive, flexible and highly therapeutic. Very few of the operations involved are of a complex nature, while much of the contributory work is unskilled, simple and easily performed by any patient, with only the elementary knowledge of how to use a shovel, such as preparing and mixing the aggregate, as well as feeding the concrete mixture to the other operators. The laying out of the finished products for setting, as well as subsequent removal from the pallets and the cleaning and oiling of the latter will also provide simple occupations for even Group I type of patients, whose promotion to the more skilled operations of the craft provides the therapeutic stepping-stone arrangement of work, so important in promoting recovery.

The existence of a sandpit in the hospital estate will also create very useful auxiliary work in providing a very essential raw material, whose purchase might otherwise be prohibitive. The work of raising the sand and gravel and grading by means of screening, with subsequent washing before use, would increase further the occupational content of this craft and thus add to the element of versatility and flexibility, so important a feature of cementcraft as a whole. It might be mentioned here that the preparation of the aggregate by thorough washing before mixing with the cement, limits the porosity of the finished products, as well as increasing their strength and solidity, well above accepted commercial standards.

(5) *Quality*. Quality refers to certain intrinsic attributes or features, proper to each handicraft, which facilitate grading to meet psychological application. Such characteristics are the various grades of complexity, ranging from simple minor to major, already described, though these qualities tend to have a sliding value in many crafts, dependent on the mode and stage of application, as well as the capacity for adjustment, already referred to under *Adaptability*. For instance, weaving may be utilized in its very simplest, as well as in its various more complicated forms and this important property of adjustment creates the sliding value mentioned. Basketry, whether in willow-work or cane-work, and many other crafts, exhibit a similar regulatory quality.

*The Economic Qualities* appertaining to each craft will also require due recognition. With the therapeutic viewpoint accorded primary attention at all times, commercial considerations must enter into the complete analysis of all therapeutic crafts. The adoption of sound business methods in dealing with the commercial requirements of O.T. departments, will necessitate close examination and study of all the qualities and factors associated with the economic and technical side of the different handicrafts.

Such economic considerations will cover the nature and qualities of (a) *the materials* and *the equipment* required for each craft. The materials available for use must be subjected to an exhaustive analysis, in regard to technical suitability and relationship to extent of costings, as well as considering questions of utility and (b) *disposal of finished products*.

(a) *Materials, Tools and Equipment* will require examination to embrace therapeutic, utility, suitability and economic considerations, so as to ensure that the arrangements for the purchase of all O.T. requisites will maintain proper and uninterrupted treatment services at all times. A proper knowledge of the nature of the many different types and qualities of materials is essential to secure a suitable selection for O.T. purposes. Likewise, in the matter of tools and equipment, the purchase of the right type of article involves a proper analysis of each item from the huge and varied ranges on offer.

(b) *The Disposal and Saleability* of the finished products will also involve suitable analysis, so as to correlate the commercial with the therapeutic side of the treatment and thus maintain proper harmony in the organisation and development of the different craft treatment services.

Crafts may be qualified generally as—(a) *Sedative* or (b) *Stimulative*, according to the quietening or elevating effect which they tend to exercise on the mental state during therapeutic application. For this reason, crafts with a soothing or sedative effect are prescribed for restless, agitated, elated, disturbed mental cases, while stimulative crafts are indicated for the retarded, stuporose, melancholic and apathetic types.

Generally speaking, crafts, whose processes consist mainly of simple, monotonous, repetitive movements, involving little or no colour effect, with drabness of both shade and design, are described as sedative, while the stimulative crafts possess a variety of processes, involving constant attention and more concentrated application, with the introduction of a variety of coloured materials and attractive designs. Simple Raffiawork or simple willow or cane basketry or simple plain weaving may be cited as examples of sedative crafts, while advanced twill weaving in colours, as well as all carpet making whether by weaving or knitting, where intricacy of coloured design is a feature, are examples of stimulative handicrafts. Strangely enough, many crafts, like some of those cited, can be regulated to produce either sedative or stimulative results, as required. For instance, weaving, of the simple, monotonous type, without colour and, consequently, sedative, may be arranged to produce stimulative effects by the introduction of both colour and design. This transformation can be achieved on the same loom, even a table loom, by the use of coloured yarns in simple or twill weaves.

Occupational therapy has also been described as (1) *Active* or (2) *Passive*, according to the patient's relationship to the immediate source of the treatment. In (1) the patient is actively engaged in the treatment and operating it for his own benefit, even though under supervision, while in (2) the patient is, in a passive manner, receiving treatment, which is being operated for his benefit by others, such as in cinema or concert shows, or team games or sports, where the patient is merely an interested spectator. Such a distinction in quality is only applicable, generally, to recreational therapy activities, if we exclude the very rare occasions when a patient is in receipt of passive treatment, when watching with interest the performance, by another patient or group of patients, of the more skilled and technical processes of a craft.

A further objective classification of crafts, concerned with location, is of importance, as it forms the basis of the division of crafts in the daily Handicraft Therapy Report Books, sample pages from which are reproduced facing page 135 and on page 136 (Figs. 10 and 11). These are classified generally, as follows:—(1) *Special Handicraft Pavilion*, (2) *Ward*, (3) *Bedside*, (4) *Utility and Technical* and (5) *General*.

### 1—*Special Handicraft Therapy Pavilion*

This, incorporating both male and female sections, is a special detached building, suitably situated at a convenient distance from the main hospital buildings. A sketch plan of such a building appears in chapter 5. In this are housed the advanced crafts, provided for Group III type of patients, such as Weaving, Basketry, Brushcraft, etc., and may or may not incorporate some of the technical sections referred to in (4) herewith. In addition, the building should include the administrative quarters for the occupational therapists on some such arrangement as shown in the sketch plan in chapter 5. This Occupational Therapy Pavilion may correctly be regarded as housing the main convalescent sections of the Occupational Therapy Department and bears somewhat the same relationship to Handicraft Therapy that the Hospital Recreational Hall bears to Recreational Therapy.

### 2—*Ward Occupations*

These refer to crafts in use in the various wards throughout the Hospital, including those availed of in the special Occupational Wards and even in the Infirmary Wards. The class-

ification and development of this type of occupation is a
necessary and essential feature of the treatment. Many patients,
for both psychological and physical reasons, cannot be submitted
for treatment outside their respective wards and special
crafts have been arranged and devised to meet the individual
needs of these patients. This necessitates a very wide grading
of occupations from the very simple kindergarten type, such
as rag-teasing, floor-polishing, sanding, paper-cutting, etc.,
for the acute as well as the more chronic deteriorated types,
up to the more advanced stage of weaving, basketry, leathercraft, etc. This range of ward crafts would include all those
classed as (1) Simple and (2) Minor complex. Major complex
occupations are rarely located in the wards as they provide
the final stages of the treatment for those who have progressed
beyond ward activities, whether by reason of convalescence
or improved skill acquired with the remission of mental
symptoms.

The development of ward occupations provides for the
application of the treatment for a very large proportion of
the patient population, as well as creating the initial stepping-
stone stages of the treatment previously referred to. Its
full extension through all wards, whether of the refractory
or chronic type, constitutes a basic condition in occupational
therapy development, even if less dramatic and spectacular
than the more highly organised special extra-ward sections.

### 3—Bedside Occupations

Bedside occupations have been specially devised to provide
treatment for those mental cases, who, by reason of physical
disease or defect, are confined to bed, whether in a temporary
or permanent capacity and when the physical condition
present does not preclude occupational treatment. Acute
illnesses and infections, particularly with pyrexia as a prominent feature, are an obvious contraindication. Prescription
cards will only be issued by the medical staff in suitable
cases. In these cases, the problem of the occupational
therapist will be governed by the horizontal or vertical
position of the patient, as well as simplicity and adaptability
of the necessary apparatus.

A highly essential equipment is an adjustable bedside table, the leaf of which can be fixed at any angle that will facilitate operation of the prescribed craft, in relation to the patient's recumbent or upright position. This table should possess special clamping devices for immobilising the material or materials to be operated on. Small table or braid looms may be so fixed and arranged to simplify the movement of the hand shuttle. Special weaving frames, of larger type that sit across the bed on uprights resting on the floor, may be provided for convalescent patients permitted to sit upright. Such patients may also engage in a variety of crafts that do not require any special apparatus, such as knotting, rake-knitting, simple raffiawork and simple basketry, etc. In the latter, the material is prepared for the patient, either in the special section arranged for the craft or in the wash-room or other suitable room off the ward, where the water and other arrangements are satisfactory.

In the matter of bedside occupations, recreations and hobbies will also enter prominently into the picture, as distinct from handicrafts. Passive and active amusements, such as painting, reading, musical programmes, philately (stamp-collecting and arranging), etc., may prove more suitable and more beneficial in certain special cases. Even specially arranged ward concerts and wireless programmes will add appreciably to the craft facilities available for all patients confined to bed. There will always be a number of chronic infirmary cases, who will avidly devour any reading material provided and for them this will prove a very important type of bedside occupation.

### 4—*The Utility and Technical Sections*

These Utility sections constitute the various upkeep and maintenance activities, which are standard in practically all mental hospitals and previously listed.

All of these Utility sections constitute craftwork of a specialised type and are each under the immediate supervision of a skilled and experienced worker, whose technical advice and assistance is available to the occupational therapist in adapting them as very special treatment centres.

### 1—*The Laundry*

This section provides utility work of a specially technical type and is staffed with a trained personnel under a Head Laundress, who supervises and assists at the more skilled and advanced parts of the many operations involved. Laundry-work constitutes occupation of a very flexible and diversified type, mainly of a sedative nature. It provides a wide range of activities, graduating in complexity from very simple to highly skilled activities, which are very adaptable for treatment purposes, because of the skilled advice and assistance always at hand. As a treatment centre, therefore, it absorbs female patients from all the three main groups into which psychotic patients are generally classified. Group I patients would be suitably catered for in the very simple operations connected with steeping of clothes, carting to washing machines and subsequently to drying machines and external drying lines and their return for ironing and finishing. All these simple manual operations are within the competency of many very regressed schizophrenic patients.

More skilled operations of a minor complex nature are available for Group II types, such as hand ironing, hand washing and preparation of the necessary laundry materials for starching, etc. The more highly skilled and complex work, associated with the operation of the various washing, ironing and drying machines, as well as electrical hand ironing, etc., will meet the needs of Group III patients. The diversified nature of laundrycraft is also exemplified by its capacity to provide individual or group therapy. Those patients who prefer individual effort may be treated separately from those who revel in teamwork and the manifold operations in the laundry provide facilities for this.

### 2—*The Kitchen*

Kitchencraft is very much akin to Laundry work because of the many varying activities in the preparation and cooking of food, involving operations, ranging from the simplest to the most complex. All these, however, are more stimulative and provide more variation in quality, though less complex in general. Kitchenwork, nevertheless, shows greater restriction in regard to the extent of skilled personnel available for supervision and in the numbers in receipt of treatment.

### 3—The Dining Halls

The refectory sections of the hospital afford treatment for quite a number of patients, particularly when associated with the preparation, as well as the distribution of the various items of food. The work, here, is more sedative than stimulative, but the variety of operations associated with the different meals maintains interest. The work too may be graded from simple scullerycraft and general cleaning and washing, to the operation of special hand machines provided for bread-cutting, washing of tableware, etc. None of the work, however, approaches a standard of major complexity, but provides sufficient variation in the many daily procedures involved to render it attractive for quite a large number of patients, both male and female. The daily repetitive nature of the work, tending towards a sedative effect, is of such a varied type from hour to hour, as to introduce a stimulative quality and thus afford treatment for a wide range of patients.

The many activities embraced in providing the daily meals for the majority of the hospital patients are under the immediate direction and supervision of a skilled and experienced nurse. These constitute the washing and cleaning of the various items of tableware and utensils, the preparation and laying of the table for the different meals, the subsequent removal of all tableware and utensils for washing and cleaning and the collection and appropriate disposal of the waste food. All this involves a good deal of transport by hand—the collecting and conveyance of all items of food from the kitchen and their proper distribution as between all tables and each position at table. There is also the general maintenance and washing of the refectories and adjoining sections of the hospital, which is carried out in the between-meal periods. The close association with food demands constant personal cleanliness, inculcating habits of neatness and tidiness, which tend to augment the therapeutic advantages of this type of craft treatment.

## 4—*The Farm, Gardens and Grounds*

These constitute three utility sections that are a standard feature in all public mental hospitals. All three sections are under the immediate supervision of a fully-trained and experienced Farm Steward who, as a general rule, is supported by an Assistant Farm Steward with similar qualifications. They are aided by an auxiliary staff of gardeners, ploughmen, herdsmen, dairymen, etc., who are available for skilled advice in the operation of their respective spheres of husbandry. All these act as special technicians in arranging therapeutical work for large groups of patients under the immediate supervision of nurses, who, by their active participation in the working details of the different sections of the treatment, may qualify as special occupational nurses.

### *The Advantages of Husbandry*

The therapeutic importance of these three sections of husbandry, all grouped under the control of the Farm Steward, may be gauged from the many special *characteristics and advantages* afforded by them as treatment centres, which are listed as follows:—

1. They provide facilities for group or individual therapy, as required. Though the activities generally are of the group type, there are special opportunities for providing individual tasks for those patients whose prescription cards emphasise individual treatment as opposed to group work.

2. There is a wide range of technical assistance and advice available, as described above. This enables those patients of limited experience in this type of craftwork, to overcome any technical obstacles that might otherwise restrict the amplitude as well as the efficacy of the treatment.

3. The work, being mainly outdoor, provides open-air treatment that may be very necessary for a number of patients, whether based on the physical grounds of health or because of claustrophobiac or other such obsessional tendencies.

4. The three sections provide a wide and varied range of

occupations, so differing in complexity as to create a veritable stepping-stone arrangement of treatment services from the very simplest type of work for the most regressed of the Group I patients to very highly skilled and complex work for the convalescent patients in Group III. This facility for providing treatment for almost every type of psychotic and psychoneurotic patient in the one section or group of allied sections, classified as husbandry, exhibits a quality of flexibility unequalled by any other type of therapeutic craft. It has, consequently, the very great advantage of absorbing the largest complement of patients in relation to the various other occupations that are accepted as standard in all fully-developed occupational therapy departments.

*The Disadvantages of Husbandry*, by way of contrast, are mainly two:—

1. Treatment is generally confined to male patients, though floriculture and other types of light gardening may be provided for female patients.

2. Weather difficulties may cause some restriction in maintaining continuous treatment, but such blank days may be offset by recreational change, usually arranged for Sabbath Days and other non-farming days.

These disadvantages do not, in any way, limit the therapeutic element, inherent in all activities associated with husbandry and the time limitations mentioned are of very little significance when related to the several advantages outlined.

The work associated with the Farm, Garden and upkeep of the hospital grounds is probably of a more varied type than that associated with any other handicraft activity. It incorporates a very wide range of complexity, covering work of both a skilled and unskilled type. Its ever-varying nature is an outstanding characteristic, comprising the manifold activities associated with dairying, including the care, feeding and milking of the herd, as well as the feeding, grooming and general guidance of the farm horses and other stock. The many and varied items of machinery involve repair and servicing, as well as utilisation for the work appropriate to each, such as, ploughing, harrowing, seed and root sowing, meadow-cutting and mowing, reaping, binding and threshing, crop-digging and general harvesting, all of which involve a good deal of cartage and general transport of farm commodities.

In addition, there are many auxiliary activities, including pig-rearing and fattening, poultry farming and all types of gardening, etc. The latter provides a most versatile range of activities, not least among which may be cited kitchen-gardening, providing for the cultivation of the manifold table vegetables required for hospital consumption. There is also the cultivation of flowers as well as fruit-gardening of all kinds. All of these open up an avenue of activities that provide a very attractive range of treatment services for suitable patients.

The care and maintenance of the hospital grounds and avenues also provide a wide range of activities that absorb quite a large number of patients. These involve the cutting and trimming of lawns with appropriate hand-machines, the cleaning, trimming and surfacing of the avenues and walks throughout the grounds; hedges, shrubs and trees require perennial attention and all activities involve a certain amount of cartage with hand-barrows and wheelbarrows, as well as the use of hand-rollers, etc. The flower-beds and rock-gardens, too, require sowing, transplanting and weeding, as well as general upkeep, in accordance with seasonal demands.

The extremely diverse and novel nature of all the manifold activities associated with farming, gardening and general husbandry, would indicate a very marked combination of both sedative and stimulative qualities in the nature of most of the activities. Consequently, the prescription requirements for farmwork and allied occupations require a very deep analysis for each type of activity to obviate placing 'a square peg in a round hole' and thus to ensure that the quality of the work prescribed is that best adapted for the psychotic condition under treatment.

### 5—The Seamstress's Department

This is another very important utility section, which, with the skilled and technical assistance of the seamstress, provides a variety of work, embracing a number of well-recognised occupational therapy crafts. Machine and hand-sewing, machine and hand-knitting, stitchcraft of all kinds, female tailoring and repair-work covering general clothing requirements, constitute a range of interesting occupations affording treatment services for quite a large number of patients. There is the added advantage that the technical knowledge and advice of the seamstress will tend to simplify treatment application for many non-skilled patients, whose prescription requirements might be restricted otherwise.

The varied nature of the work associated with the manufacture of the general clothing requirements of the hospital, both patients and staff, is both stimulative and sedative and proper analysis in prescribing any individual craft housed in this section is essential for this reason.

### 6—*The Tradeshops*

These, including the Bakery, comprise a varied range of utility sections, constituting a wide medley of activities, both skilled and unskilled. All these technical sections are a standard feature of the large mental hospitals and are each in the charge of a professional tradesman. The skilled advice and assistance of the latter in the operation of his respective craft, as in other utility sections, reinforces the therapeutic element, even for the non-skilled patients submitted for treatment.

Chief among these centres are (a) *The Carpenter's Shop*, (b) *The Painter's Shop*, (c) *The Shoemaker's Shop*, (d) *The Plasterer's Shop*, including such allied activities as *roof-slating, masonry cementcraft, etc.*, (e) *The Upholsterer's Shop*, (f) *The Tailor's Shop* and (g) *The Bakery*.

(a) *Carpentry and Woodworking* of all kinds involve such a wide range of activities and of such a diversified nature, that it should be possible to create a number of separate treatment units. These latter units can be organised in the general woodworking centre, where the hospital Carpenter would be available for technical advice and assistance in each unit when required. These units, as woodworking sub-sections, would operate such crafts as:—Turnery, furniture manufacture, wooden toy manufacture, manufacture of wooden articles required in other units of the handicraft therapy department, as well as in the hospital generally, etc.    A special analysis of woodcraft is detailed in a later chapter.

(b) *The Painter's Shop* provides a suitable centre for all forms of paintcraft and allied activities, such as the preparation and mixing of paints in the different colours, as required, the preparation of various stains in both oil and water, as well as the manufacture of putty and cutting of sheet glass of all kinds for subsequent glazing.  In this centre arrangements may be made for finishing many articles completed in other occupational therapy sections, by enamelling in paint or staining with varnish finish.  Provision may also be made for the various operations connected with polish-finishing, whether of the french, wax or oil variety.  The close association of most of the work with that of the woodworking centre, suggests that both centres might, with advantage, be placed as contiguous as possible.

(c) *The Shoemaker's Shop* provides a leathercraft centre which may be regarded as the least important of the utility sections, from the therapeutic point of view, for the following reasons:—

1. The craft has a rather restrictive quality from the point of view of application, as the work is mainly of the skilled type and can only be prescribed for unskilled patients in very exceptional cases, such as the case mentioned in chapter 5.

2. The work involved is extremely monotonous and of the repetitive type and, consequently, strongly sedative and thus further restricted in application.

3. It is not a suitable centre for developing the more novel and more stimulative type of fancy leathercraft, which is generally operated in the special O.T. Pavilion.

(d) *The Plasterer's Shop* opens up a number of attractive occupations, associated with the work of the Plasterer, which involve a wide range of many dissimilar activities, chief of which is cementcraft, both plain and coloured, which has been described in detail in the early part of this chapter.

Roof-slating and tiling, as well as plastering of all kinds, both indoor and outdoor, may be regarded as the skilled activities in this section, which are characterised by the same restriction in application as prevails in the Shoemaker's shop. Masonry, stone-building and bricklaying, when not supervised by a tradesman, skilled solely in one or other of these crafts, may be included in the Plasterer's section as being closely allied. While the skilled portions of these three crafts may provide treatment for a very limited number of patients, the volume of auxiliary work in each will open up therapeutic employment for quite a number of patients which is mainly of the outdoor variety.

(e) *The Upholsterer's Shop*, which is, generally, also under the supervision of a skilled tradesman, provides therapeutic occupation, which has the great advantage that there is scarcely any activity in the course of the work involved, that is not within the competence of any Grade 3 patient. While it is characterised, mainly, as an utility section, providing an important repair service for the hospital generally, it is capable of development, in conjunction with the furniture-making unit of the wood-working centre, by extending its activities to the production of finished articles, whether for hospital replacements or for outside or other disposal.

(f) *The Tailor's Shop* is the male side counterpart of the Seamstress's department in the female side of the hospital, being concerned with the production of the male clothing, mainly the outer garments—the jacket, vest, pants, etc. The work is, chiefly, that associated with stitchcraft in trimming and making the male suitings from the tweeds woven in the special occupational therapy pavilion. The skilled side of the work will provide rather sedative occupation for a limited number of patients, but the general repair of the clothing, whether in the shop or the wards, will provide a substantial amount of work for an additional number of suitable patients, whose prescription requirements may suggest this type of sedative work.

(g) *The Bakery* is an utility section in operation in all those hospitals, where the bread requirements are not purchased on outside contracts and creates employment for a rather limited quota of patients. The demands of the hospital may necessitate the use of machinery for some of the operations, but a good deal of handwork provides suitable indoor occupation, even if limited in scope.

### 7—*The Engineering Department*

This section comprises a number of units, involving many different crafts, such as boiler-stoking, plumbing, pipe-fitting, machine-shop work and general metalcraft, as well as forge work and general hospital engineering. The entire department is supervised by a skilled Engineer with a number of assistants, comprising Stokers, Fitters, Plumbers, Electricians, etc., and each of these, in his own unit, provides occupation for a number of patients, which can be regulated on a therapeutic basis.

All the crafts concerned, though largely skilled, are of a more stimulative type than most of the trades discussed. The skilled nature of the majority of the operations in each unit is not beyond the grasp of many Grade III patients, but there is a very substantial range of unskilled activities in all units, which provides therapeutic occupation of a stimulative type.

In the Engineering department it is possible to open up a special metalcraft unit, which, in addition to effecting machinery and other repairs, will afford facilities for the manufacture of many iron and steel commodities required in many different parts of the hospital, such as steel gates and railings, steel frames, for many purposes, etc.

This general analysis of the crafts covers the whole general range of occupations that are in operation in all large mental hospitals. It is necessary, however, to analyse, in more detail, some of the more important crafts, that are a standard feature of every fully developed occupational therapy department. This constitutes special craft analysis, which is dealt with in the ensuing chapters.

# CHAPTER XIV.

## SPECIAL CRAFT ANALYSIS

### Willowcraft, Canecraft, etc.

THE QUESTION of Craft Analysis for the purpose of occupational treatment has been covered in a general way in the preceding chapter and consideration must now be given to the problem of analysing the most important of the individual occupations in a detailed and specific manner. This is known as *Individual Craft Analysis* and must, as such, be governed by the various principles and rules of guidance laid down in the previous general analysis.

This special analysis of the major handicrafts is essential and must include a detailed examination, covering every aspect, whether psychological, physical, technical, or commercial, so as to assess in a comprehensive way, the therapeutic and other qualities of these crafts. The fulfilment of the prescription recommendations in each individual case submitted for treatment can only be suitably achieved through the knowledge derived from such exhaustive analysis. It facilitates, not only the selection of a suitable craft, but it simplifies adjustment of the grade of activity in the craft selected, to suit the condition to be treated. It conduces to scientific application of occupational treatment and thus ensures maximum therapeutic results. It is only by means of such detailed analysis that the stepping-stone arrangement of O.T., so necessary for universal application, can be organised.

It is not possible, within the limitations of a text such as this, to include an analysis of every possible therapeutic occupation and preference must, of necessity, be accorded to some of the more important crafts, which have been described as *Major Crafts*. The actual rating, as to importance, of these major crafts may be one of purely personal opinion, but their order, as to discussion, should not affect the extent or the value of the analyses concerned.

For similar reasons, it is not practicable or feasible to discuss all the technical details with regard to the working and operation of each craft, except in so far as may be necessary for the elaboration of any particular point or points in any individual analysis. Complete details as to the various processes involved in the operation of all these crafts will be found in the many appropriate craft books published, quite a number of which is scheduled in the appendix at the end of the text and a close study of most of these is essential for a fuller and more complete understanding of the analyses of the crafts discussed. With regard to the problem of craft selection generally, the eminent American authority, Dr. William Rush Dunton, Jr., makes the following pertinent reference in his interesting work—*Prescribing Occupational Therapy:*—

'Relative to the choice of crafts, it sometimes simplifies our problem if we remember that all handwork or craft activities are grouped around six materials; that is, Wood, Metal, Paper, Textiles, Clay and Leather. The place where they are to be used (bed, ward, shop, outdoor) may influence our choice and the desired physical or mental result perhaps may be attained with several of them.'

The following crafts are listed for special analyses, as constituting the chief crafts, which should be included as special treatment centres in any complete Occupational Therapy Scheme. There are generally standard crafts in the O.T. departments of practically all the large mental hospitals and their rating in order of importance is based, among a number of other considerations, mainly on the element of universality in the extent of application:—(1) *Willowcraft and Canecraft*, including *Basketry*, (2) *Woodworking*, (3) *Weaving*, (4) *Cementcraft*, (5) *Papercraft*, including *Printing and Bookbinding*, (6) *Brushcraft*, (7) *Husbandry*, (8) *Stitchcraft*, (9) *Wirecraft*, (10) *Rug and Matmaking*, (11) *Metalwork*, (12) *Dyecraft*, (13) *Upholstery*, (14) *Pottery*, (15) *Leathercraft*,

(16) *Design and Paintcraft* and (17) *Crafts in Waste Materials.*

The first three of these major crafts have been selected for special analysis in the order listed and the method and arrangement of the analysis adopted can be followed in the case of any of the remaining major occupations listed, *mutata mutandis.*

(1) *Willowcraft and Canecraft (Basketry):* Handwork in willow or 'osiers,' usually associated with basketmaking, is regarded as one of the oldest crafts in the world, dating back very many centuries before the birth of Christ. The subsequent use of more pliable materials, such as the various types of cane, raffia, Chinese Grass (seagrass), rush, and more latterly plastic materials, has extended the scope of the craft to many other developments additional to basketry, such as the manufacture of trays, furniture, lampshades, as well as chair-seating, etc. Apart from this element of flexibility, it has many other commendable qualities, which give it the primary position among the entire range of therapeutic crafts.

Examination and analysis of the craft will be considered under the following heads: (1) *Qualities*, both subjective and objective, (2) *Economic*, dealing with (a) equipment, (b) materials and (c) sales, (3) *Technical*, covering the various operations and activities met with, (4) *Psychological*, (5) *Physical*, (6) *Advantages* and (7) *Disadvantages.*

## 1—*Qualities*

(A) *Adaptability:* This is a special quality of adjustment, which is more prominent in basketry than in any other handicraft, because it can be adapted for the application of treatment to most types of patients covering all three grades previously referred to. In other words, the movements associated with the work can be regulated from the very simple type, such as the single weave (randing) on timber or plywood bases, to the use of more elaborate weaves, such as slewing, different types of waling, etc., with the substitution of woven bases for timber ones. The complexity of the work may be increased also by the introduction of more intricate designs, by way of more elaborate shapes, as well as in the making of more difficult projects, as in the case of reed furniture, table lamps, etc. These latter would only be within the competence of some of the Grade III patients.

Willowwork and concomitant activities are, accordingly, highly adaptable in their wide extent of application, meeting the needs of practically every grade of patient and thus embracing a high therapeutic content. It can also be adjusted to suit the physical capacity present. Light as well as heavy projects can be arranged as required and the element of fatigue may, in this way, be avoided or, at least, restricted to the minimum. The simpler forms of cane and raffia basketry are examples of work of a light type, while the manufacture of laundry baskets and very large hampers, as well as the more bulky items of furniture, constitutes the heavier work in this craft.

(B) *Subjective Effect:* The craft has the additional regulatory quality in that it can be adjusted to produce either (1) a *sedative* or (2) a *stimulative* effect and, consequently, can be arranged to suit the mental condition submitted for treatment as distinct from the mental or intellectual capacity present, which would influence the complexity of the work prescribed, as detailed under (A) *Adaptability.*

(1) The simple types of single weaving or randing on wooden bases, whether in raffia or cane in the absence of colour, because of the monotonous repetition involved, would have a quieting or *sedative* effect on the restless, agitated or hyperactive patients under treatment.

(2) The introduction of colours of more advanced and more difficult weaves, with greater intricacy in design or shape, would create a *stimulative* effect, which is required for the depressed or apathetic type of patient. This is easily achieved in willow and cane work, even when it is necessary, in addition, to make suitable adjustments with regard to the complexity of the work to meet the capacity of performance in the patient concerned.

(C) *Objective Qualities:* (a) *Complexity.* Owing to the possibility of adjustment already referred to, the craft embraces all grades of complexity, from the very simple to highly complex projects, as detailed under (A) *Adaptability,* consequently, basketry and allied activities will provide suitable treatment for all grades of patients from the very lowest and regressed type right up to the highest grade, including the convalescent cases, where the special prescription requirements are so indicated. This stepping-stone arrangement of treatment services, referred to previously in the text, in the general arrangement of the different occupations, is exemplified here in the one craft, which permits of a complete range of complexity from the very simplest to the most complex project. Such an arrangement, present perhaps only to the same extent in woodworking, adds an additional therapeutic factor to the already very high treatment value of this craft.

(b) *Flexibility:* This craft, as already detailed, is highly flexible in the mode and extent of application. It provides treatment for practically every type of mental condition, because of the possibility of adjustment previously discussed, in regard to both complexity and to the subjective effect required, whether sedative or stimulative. In addition, adjustment is permissible to suit the physical capacity of the patient by providing light or heavy work, as required.

(c) *Novelty and Variety* in the work is also exemplified by the wide range of activities that may be carried on, not only in the manufacture of the many different types of baskets, such as shopping baskets, work and needle baskets, cycle baskets, laundry baskets, hampers, fishing baskets, etc., but also in the production of various other articles made from willow, cane, etc., such as reed furniture, cane trays, table lamps, lampshades, etc.

(d) *Utility:* The many hospital requirements in baskets of all types, as well as in the associated products mentioned already, give this occupation a very strong utilitarian quality, which adds to its flexibility by maintaining a continuity in treatment services, which may not be possible in the case of most of the other therapeutic occupations. Many crafts may provide only intermittent occupation because of the possibility of over-production leading to difficulties in disposal. Basketry and allied work, because of the high utility content, is not so restricted and this provides an additional reason for its primal rating among the other therapeutic occupations.

## 2—Economic

Commercial viewpoints, as already stated, should not enter as a primary consideration into the recommendation of any occupation, but any economic advantages possessed by an O.T. craft should increase its rating value over other occupations of equal therapeutic content. *Willow-work* presents many economic points of advantage that place it far above all other crafts. These are discussed under (a) *Equipment*, (b) *Materials* and (c) *Disposal of Products*.

(a) *Equipment:* Equipment is of the very minimum in comparison with most other occupations. Apart from a tank, made of iron or in cement aggregate, for steeping the willows or cane to facilitate working, the following inexpensive tools and equipment are required: (1) *Hand-knife* or *Pen-knife* for general purposes, (2) *Picking Knife* for cutting off any surplus projecting ends of willows or canes in an otherwise completed basket, (3) different types of *Bodkins*, the *Shell Bodkin* or straight type to facilitate staking or cramming by forming a passage for the insertion of the stakes or crams (used in finishing plain borders) and the *Bent Bodkin*, which is necessary for insertion of handle-bows into the curved sides of a basket. The straight bodkin, which is somewhat similar to a bradawl in shape, may also be used instead of the latter in the centre of the basket bottom to keep it in position and still allow it to revolve while weaving, (4) a *Shears*, which is merely a small pruning shears, is also included in the equipment, (5) a *Rapping Iron*, which may be described as the basket-maker's hammer, is used for levelling off and closing in the weaves, as well as for any hammering that may be necessary. It may be on a light or heavy type to suit the work on hand, (6) *Work Boards*, which are simple, small wooden planks, either of the (a) flat horizontal type for heavy work or (b) with a batten attached beneath one end to create a sloping position for working on the smaller types of baskets. These work boards are used for circular weaving. In the case of rectangular baskets, it will be necessary to use (7) a *Screw-Block* when making the bottoms or covers of these baskets, so as to immobilise the uprights in position while weaving, (8) *Round-nosed Pliers*, as well as *a pair of Pincers and Side-Cutters*, are also used in the course of the work, as required.

For *Skein Work*, which uses strips of split willow (skeins) for making light types of baskets, such as letter baskets, as well as for lapping basket handles, etc., a few special tools are required for the preparation of the skeins, as follows:— (1) A *Cleave*, which splits each willow into uniform strips, is generally of the three-way type, forming three skeins in the process of splitting. Four-way Cleaves are also available, but little used, as they require special experience for successful manipulation. Even the three-way type introduces an element of higher complexity in stripping the willows successfully, so as to produce skeins of uniform size, because the process is one of splitting and not cutting. (2) A *Shave* is also used for removing the pith of the skeins and thus thinning them to requirements. An additional tool, known as (3) the *Upright* is also used when it is necessary to reduce the width of the skeins to narrow and uniform sizes for exceedingly fine and delicate work and, in particular, for *Listing*. This is a special form of raised ornamentation of lapped handles by using what are described as listing-skeins, skeins, which are lapped around an additional single whole-rod, known as a leader, placed on top of the original handle bow.

Skein work generally is of two types: (1) *Flat-Skein work* and (2) *Edge-Skein work*. The former, which is not in general use, for economic reasons mainly, shows the skeins placed flat against each other as opposed to edge-skein work, where the skeins do not lap, but are placed edge to edge, which means more rapid weaving, using lesser material, though the result is inferior. While the preparation of skeins may demand more technique and experience and thus restrictive in application, the resultant thinning of the original willows renders them easy to handle and manipulate. This widens the scope of the craft in its application for simple weaving projects, as well as for the various types of lapping associated with willowcraft, such as covering of basket handles, legs of wicker furniture, etc.

(b) *Materials:* Materials for basketry and associated activities are derived mainly from the two species of willows, *Salix Triandra* and *Salix Purpurea*, the latter providing the small types of 'rods' known as Dicky Meadows or Red Bud and the former producing a larger rod, described as Black Maul and also a smaller type called Pomeranian, all being usually one year shoots. The very heavy rods, called 'sticks' or 'osiers,' generally of two or three years' growth, used for chair frames and large hampers, may also be produced from a coarser species of willow, called *Salix Viminalis*.

Basket Willows can be cultivated in suitable land on the hospital farm by planting cuttings about 12 inches long from rods in the green at any time during the period between October and the following April. These are placed in parallel rows about 18 inches apart, with about 12 to 15 inches separating each cutting, which is placed 2 or 3 inches above ground, with the buds looking upwards. The first crop cut is not used, being unsuitable, but the cutting off improves the next crop. The rods cut from the willow 'beds' are known as 'Green Whole-stuff' and, when allowed to dry by storing, are called 'Brown.' The latter, when peeled, are known as 'White.' If the green rods are boiled before peeling, they are known as 'Buff,' because of the golden brown staining caused by the penetration of the tannic acid in the bark.

Other materials, such as Cane, Raffia, Chinese Grass (Seagrass), Rush and Straw Plait, as well as artificial and plastic substitutes, are also availed of in this craft, most of which introduces colour, as well as simplifying manipulation and thus facilitating the extension of the work to the female sections of the hospital. Cane used in basketry is of four kinds: (1) *Whole Cane*, which is only used for making coal baskets and other heavy baskets that have to be subjected to very hard wear and tear. (2) *Chair Cane*, which is simply the hard, polished skin of whole cane cut into skeins and used for seating chairs, as well as lapping basket handles, legs of wicker or cane furniture, etc. (3) *Pulp Cane*, also known

as *Centre* or *pith*, as it is made from the centre of rotten
canes from which the skin has been removed for (2) above.
It is, accordingly, available in a wide range of thicknesses,
from $1\frac{1}{2}$ mm. in diameter, known as size 1 up to size 20,
which is 8 mm. in diameter. It is also available as flat or
strip cane of varying substances. *Pulp* or *Centre cane*,
which is available in several different lengths up to even
16 feet, is very easily manipulated and suitable, therefore,
for female patients. It is, consequently, much more adaptable
for light, fancy work, even though, in its raw state, it does
not possess the glossy finish of white or buff willows. It
can, however, be finished by staining and varnishing or by
coating with good quality enamel paint. Although pulp
cane is easily dyed in colours, the result is very fugitive,
even when varnished over. (4) *Split Cane* is also used for
weaving and lapping and is derived from the whole cane by
splitting down the middle and shaving afterwards to the
substance required.

Raffia, Seagrass, Rush and Straw are also plaited and used
in basketry to create a fancy, attractive finish and they may
be used in conjunction with Pulp cane to introduce special
colour effect.

(c) *Disposal of Products:* The ready market for baskets
of all types, wicker and cane furniture, etc., particularly
owing to the many different types of articles that are possible
of manufacture, gives this craft a very strong precedence
over all others in the matter of products disposal. This is
particularly so in the case of the mental hospital where the
basket and associated products required will be met by a
very high percentage of the annual O.T. output. The balance
of the products sold externally will, as a general rule, provide
for continuity in operation of the craft, as detailed under
(d) *Utility* (p.215). Some outstanding economic advantages
in this craft are (a) the limited and, consequently, inexpensive
equipment required, consisting of a small number of light
and easily obtained tools, which reduces the supervisory
and precautionary measures that have to be considered
in the therapeutic handling of all crafts and (b) the facility
for producing the chief raw material—the willow rods,

as well as their purchase at very little cost from numerous vendors, who cultivate 'beds' or 'holts' on a large scale in most countries. The other materials also listed, such as Cane, Raffia, etc., can also be bought at proportionately reasonable prices and there is no limit to supplies under normal conditions.

### 3—Technical

The operations involved in Willowcraft and allied occupations are based on the simple weave—crossing the weft under and over the fixed stakes or warps, or, alternately on either side of them, depending on whether the stakes are positioned vertically or horizontally while being worked, This is known as *Randing* or *Single Weaving* and used to fill up the sides of the main body of the work. This may be light when the weft rods nearly touch each other and are not packed tightly together as in *close randing*. *Double Weaving*, known as Pairing, may be described as a type of randing, using two rods instead of one. These two rods, in addition to each being worked alternately in front and behind different stakes, pass alternately under and over each other between each stake. Where two or more rods are used and passed together alternately behind and in front of the same stakes, each rod occupying an unchanged position, either above or below its comrade, this is known as *Slewing*, being either two-rod or three-rod, as the case may be. It is simply a form of randing where two or three rods are used in the same manner as if they were one rod, lying vertically one immediately above the other. Rods used for slewing must be thinner than those used for randing, to compensate for the extra pressure on the stakes caused by two or three rods as against the single rod in randing.

A special weave, known as *Waling*, worked with three or more rods, on the same principle as pairing, is used for both its reinforcing and appearance value. When used at the bottom of the sides of a basket, it is referred to as *Upsetting*, as it 'sets up' the stakes. The three or four rods used are worked alternately over and under each other, each rod in turn passing in front of two, three or more stakes and behind one. Reversing this by taking each rod in front of one stake and behind the next two or three (the latter in the case of a four-rod wale) will create the wale on the inside of the basket, as against the more usual external wale.

A special effect, though not strictly a special type of weave, is created by what is described as *Fitching*. This is merely a form of open-work in basketry and may be straight or cross, the latter so-called where the bye-stakes (the lighter stakes inserted on each side of the main stakes after upsetting) cross each other in an x-shaped fashion between each pair of main stakes. The actual fitch, which maintains the open-work immediately underneath, is merely a reverse type of pairing, where two rods are worked alternately under and over each other and passing on the opposite sides of each stake. When the two rods pass under and over each other twice between each stake, making a double turn, it is known as *Jack Fitching*. This latter may be necessary where there is extra space between the stakes, as a single turn fitch would not make for firmness.

*Borderwork and Handlework* introduce very special types of weaving, involving both simple and advanced operations in both cane and willowcraft. There are five different types of borders, each type exhibiting further individual variations, as follows:—

(a) *The Scallop* or *Open Border* is the very simplest type, but only suitable for small articles, which will not be subjected to hard wear and is, consequently, used more for its artistic effect, as in the case of glass-holders, table mats, dolls' furniture, etc.

(b) *The Track Border* is the simplest of the closed type of border and is used for small baskets. It may be of the single stake or double stake type and is easily taught to those patients who may find difficulty in coping with the more intricate and complex borders.

(c) *The Plain Border* may be of the Two-Rod, Three-Rod, Four-Rod or Five-Rod type and, in each, may be either of the single or double variety, referred to as the 'behind-one' or the 'behind-two' variety, according as each stake is brought down behind one stake or two stakes.

(d) *The Plait Border* is so called because of the plaited effect. It admits of quite a number of variations, dependent on whether two rods are worked or three rods and even by the number of pairs or threes that may be used. Variation is also effected by working the pairs or threes in front of two stakes instead of one, etc.

(e) *The Rope Border*, as the name implies, gives a corded or rope effect and may be varied by the insertion of extra rods, creating a stouter twist in the border.

*Handlework:* Basket handles are generally of two chief kinds, either (a) *Cross Handles* or (b) *Small Handles*. The former, so-called because they cross from one side of the basket border to the other and the latter being a small, single-grip type of handle erected on one side of the basket. Each of these types of handles may be either (1) *Lapped*, as referred to already under skein-work, or (2) *Roped*. This latter variety may be either of the twisted-rod or whole-rod type.

Handles may also be of the *single-rod* or *double-rod type*, according as they are made from one or two rods. A plaited type of handle is also made with three or more pairs of rods or with nine or more single rods. *Listing*, already referred to, is a form of ornamentation of lapped handles. *Ring and D-shaped Drop Handles* are also used on baskets. The former, which may be either of the plaited or twisted type, are attached to the basket with a small twisted loop. The D-shaped drop handle is skein-covered with the straight portion hinged on to the basket by means of two small loops.

There are many other technical operations associated with the many crafts allied to basketry, additional to those described, the analysis of which, for reasons of space, cannot be discussed here and reference must be had to appropriate craft books for that purpose. For instance, *Raffiawork*, which covers a wide range of interesting and useful products, though concerned with similar weaving operations as in basketry, includes additional activities, associated with wrapping, plaiting, twisting, stitching of varied kinds (Diamond, Chain, Hungarian, Fishbone, Satin, Cretan, Coral, etc., etc.), knotting, embroidering, etc.

#### 4—*Psychological*

Considerations of a psychological nature must enter into craft selection for the occupational treatment of mental conditions. Chief among these are (a) *nursing precautions and supervisory responsibilities,* as well as (b) *relationship of the craft to the mental processes aroused.*

(a) In willow-work and associated crafts, *supervisory precautions* are reduced to the minimum. The limited number and the nature of the tools, required in basketry weaving, eliminate the possibility of suicide and injury and render the work suitable for depressed patients. For this reason, supervisory demands are reduced in this type of craft and the extent of therapeutic application is increased.

(b) (1) *The Interest* aroused by the work is of maximum content, because of the unique flexibility of the craft, arising from its adaptability in application to all grades of patients and the regulatory quality present, which enables the nature of the operation to be varied by the introduction of colour, new weaves, differing shapes in projects, etc.

(2) *Attention* does not require marked concentration in the simpler, sedative projects, but, where necessary, increase in concentration can be effected by the introduction of more complex weaves and designs. This deliberate arrangement of focusing attention and increasing concentration may be essential to promote stimulative effect. It also tends to encourage the prevention of work errors and thus achieve the maximum project results, with consequent emotional satisfaction leading to the best therapeutic effect.

#### 5—*Physical*

*Fatigue:* Physical, as well as mental, can be adequately controlled in many ways—(a) *Posture* can be varied to reduce the fatigue element by arranging the work for the sitting, standing or even recumbent position. The complexity of the projects undertaken can be adjusted to suit the mental and physical needs in each individual case.

(b) *The heavy or overactive features* encountered in some of the operations may be altered to lighter and less energetic types of work, whenever the danger signal of fatigue makes its appearance. Individual requirements in these respects will be dealt with by suitable prescription recommendations or alterations, when necessary.

(c) *Eye Strain* is reduced to the minimum because of the generally coarse nature of the materials used and the easily discernible elements in the various constituents of the different operations connected with the craft. This increases the extent of application, owing to its suitability for all those suffering from eye defects and, particularly, for senile cases.

(d) *The noiseless nature of the work* generally tends to prevent the irritation that might arise from the excessive noises associated with many other handicrafts. This element of quietness adds to the sedative nature of the work generally and reduces any tendency towards the development of early fatigue.

## 6—*Advantages*

The advantages, which give Willowcraft, Basketry, etc., such a high rating among the therapeutic handicrafts, may be summarised under a number of heads, as follows:—

(a) There is an unusually high degree of *adaptability*, providing suitable occupation for all grades of mental cases, due to the wide range of *complexity* from the most simple weaving operations to the most complex projects in both weaves and design. Light and heavy work can also be adjusted to meet individual physical requirements.

(b) The exceptionally marked element of *flexibility*, revealed in the extent of adaptability described, is further emphasised by the novelty and variety of the work involved in its manifold activities, as well as the facility to change from sedative to stimulative projects and vice versa. This increases the extent of application to cover all types of mental states and diseases, as well as all three grades of patients. No other therapuetic craft exhibits such a degree of flexibility.

(c) The *psychological* advantages of the craft are exhibited by (1) *the minimum demands on supervisory responsibilities*, due to the nature and very small number of tools required for the more general weaving operations. Cutting and similar dangerous tools are not essential for the latter. (2) *Interest* in the work is maintained by the possibility of introducing variety and novelty through the wide range of activities and diverse projects available, because of the flexibility of the craft already described. (3) *Attention and concentration* can be regulated to meet the stimulative or sedative needs of the condition requiring treatment and thus improve on final results. The emotional pride and satisfaction aroused by such high standards of achievement, through proper concentration of attention, tends to secure the maximum therapeutic advantages. The flexibility and adaptability of the craft gives it a primal rating in this respect.

(d) The *physical* advantages are exhibited in (1) *the wide range of joint movements* that may be brought into play as required in the orthopaedic and other surgical fields. These cover *flexion* and *extension* of the finger, wrist, elbow and shoulder joints, as well as forearm *pronation* and *supination* and *circumduction* of wrist and shoulder joints, with a certain amount of *abduction, adduction* and *rotation* of the shoulder joints. There is also brought into play, particularly in the heavier projects, a good deal of *spinal flexion* and *extension,* as well as chest expansion. The emphasis on any one type of movement or set of movements, in accordance with individual prescription demands, may be secured by introducing the type of activity which incorporates the appropriate joint movements that require to be encouraged. (2) The *work in the craft is mainly non-fatiguing,* with the minimum of *eye-strain* and the absence of any irritating noises or sounds that might prove a contraindication. The varied nature of the light and heavy work available provides for suitable prescription in individual cases to offset the possibility of *fatigue.*

(e) Another important advantage is the *suitability of the craft for all ages and sexes.* The lighter types of work in cane basketry and other canecraft projects are very suitable for females and are featured in the female sections of most O.T. departments. These light, non-fatiguing operations in cane and similar easily-handled materials, can also be adjusted to provide therapeutic occupation for seniles, where the individual prescription requirements in each case would be the paramount consideration. The work can also be adjusted to meet the prescription needs of male adults of varying ages, where the heavier and more difficult projects may prove more suitable. The craft also permits of adjustments to provide therapeutic occupation for juveniles and children.

(f) The work involved in the various operations associated with the craft has also the added advantage in that it can be *adapted* to provide ward and bedside treatment, as well as at the special centre, where the various activities of the craft are housed. Bedside operations, however, may have to be restricted to the lighter types of canecraft.

(g) The *economic* advantages of the handicraft are also of importance and help to increase the rating value, so long as therapeutic considerations are not affected thereby. In this respect, Willowcraft and similar activities present qualities, which constitute them a very definite first among all the major O.T. crafts, whether from the standpoint of equipment, materials or utility and sales. These have already been discussed in detail under the special objective qualities associated with the utility and economic side of the work and need not be repeated here.

### 6—*Disadvantages*

The *disadvantages* connected with the craft are of the very minimum in comparison with other major O.T. activities and, in this negative manner, increase its already established primal rating value. These may be listed as follows:—

(a) The projects are mainly of an *individualistic* nature and, consequently, group therapy is restricted to the larger and heavier operations in the craft.

(b) A distinct disadvantage is the *absence of treatment facilities for lower limb joint abnormalities* in all the different activities of the craft, because of the immobilisation of these joints during practically all the operations involved. This partially restricts the therapeutic value of the craft in the orthopaedic and surgical field.

(c) The craft is also subject to *restriction in the treatment of tubercular conditions*, mainly in the phthisical cases, dependent on whether they are ambulant, semi-ambulant or confined to bed. Only the lighter types of projects may be prescribed and even these may only be suitable for the quiescent and convalescent cases. The damp nature of the materials may also prove a further contraindication in the treatment of tubercular cases.

(d) Willow-work, because of the equipment required for steeping and also steaming the osiers, *may be unsuitable for general hospitals* and similar institutions. Reed or cane, as well as raffia and such like materials, can, however, be substituted.

(e) Some objection may also be advanced to the *relatively high cost* of canes, as against willow rods, and the extent of waste, This is offset, however, by the greater facility in the handling of cane, as well as the more finished appearance of cane products, leading to quicker disposal, thus tending to solve the problem of over-production that might, otherwise, interrupt the continuity of the craft for treatment purposes.

In a general summing-up, therefore, it is clearly established that, from the extent of advantages offered and the relatively few and not very important disadvantages cited, Willowcraft, Canecraft and allied activities do stand out as the first and most important major activity available as a therapeutic occupation. The element of flexibility and adaptability in the craft, as well as the wide range and novelty of its activities, as well as many other features, not the least of which is the simplicity and ease in organising the craft, establish its exceedingly high rating value.

# CHAPTER XV.
## SPECIAL CRAFT ANALYSIS
### WOODCRAFT

(2) *Woodworking* covers a wide range of operations in the use of timber as a raw material, which have been differentiated into what are regarded as separate skilled trades, such as *Carpentry, Joinery, Turnery, Furniture-manufacture, Toy-making,* etc., and a number of auxiliary activities like *Carving, Fretwork* and *Whittling.* The working of timber as a handicraft is probably one of the oldest among the earliest known crafts and the construction of Noah's Ark comes immediately to mind in this respect. The fact that there are well over a hundred different types of trees growing in various parts of the world, with predominance of individual types in certain specified countries, explains the universality in the use of timber covering every part of the globe.

The widely differing properties of many timbers, whether in hardness, porosity, density, graining, fragility, cohesive force, toughness, colour, flexibility, susceptibility to worm infestation, expansibility, facility for polishing, resistance to water, heat and weather, freedom from knots, etc., are an indication of the multiplicity of uses that wood is and has been subjected to in all climes and in every age since the creation of mankind. These varieties in quality explain, too, the development of the many skilled activities, differing in production results, but having the common bond in the use of timber as the main raw material. These manifold activities in woodworking have resulted in such a multitudinous range of products, even within each individual skilled activity, that it is nigh impossible to make any satisfactory listing that would give even a pretence of inclusiveness. The vast majority of both heavy and light industries, the world over, is inseparably connected with the use of timber, in some form or another, in the constructive processes involved. Such widely differing activities as shipbuilding, house construction and incidental operations, manufacture of transport requirements, whether on land, sea or in the air, are an indication of the widespread use of timber, whether the emphasis is based on geographical or functional grounds.

*Woodworking* as a therapeutic craft may be classified therefore as follows:—

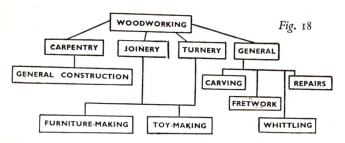

*Fig.* 18

*Carpentry* is distinguished from *Joinery* as referring to general architectural construction, mainly outdoor, the latter, with *Turnery*, being concerned in the manufacture of various utility products, chiefly indoor, such as the making of all kinds of furniture, toys, boxes, etc., while general woodworking activities, not classified under the three main previous heads, would include *wood-carving* of all kinds, *fretwork*, machine and hand and the very simple craft of penknife *whittling*, as well as repair work.

The analysis of the craft will be discussed under the same arrangement of headings as previously.

### 1—*Qualities*

(a) *Psychological: Woodworking* can be so regulated as to produce either a (1) *Sedative* or (2) *Stimulative* effect to suit the mental state or condition under treatment. Although the craft is mainly of the stimulative type, involving a variety of movements, tools, designs, colours, etc., operations involving simple repetitive movements, mainly associated with individual tools, can be organised, such as sanding, simple sawing, chiselling, simple hammering, etc. More usually, woodcraft projects, covering as they do such a relatively large range of activities, individually involving the use of many widely differing tools, achieve a stimulative effect, often in the absence of either colour changes or even intricate or elaborate designs. Woodworking, in this respect, possesses a versatility, not equalled even by basketry, though this may be offset by the restriction in application arising from the nature and proportionately greater number of tools embraced in its many diverse types of operations. As against this, most individual woodcraft projects provide a greater range of treatment services, absorbing substantially more patient personnel than in the production of willowcraft or canecraft articles.

### (B) Objective Qualities

(a) *Range of complexity:* Woodworking of all kinds provides a complete stepping-stone arrangement in degrees of complexity, from the very simplest operations involved in hand-sanding, simple hammering, planing, sawing, etc., to the most elaborate and intricate forms of carving and joint construction. All woodworking operations and craft projects may, accordingly, be graphed to indicate the degree of complexity involved and this leads to a high degree of *Adaptability.*

(b) The quality of *Adaptability* is a prominent feature of woodcraft as a therapeutic occupation. The multiplicity of operations and work projects in the use of timber render the craft highly adaptable for treatment application to embrace all three grades of mental cases. There are many and varied movements of the simple repetitive type within the competence of the most deteriorated and regressed type of patient. Such operations include the hand sanding of small and simple articles, ranging from a small batten to a completed but not very elaborate toy, the preliminary or rough planing of material required for any proposed projects, as well as the preliminary cutting by handsaw of the smaller portions of material so prepared, etc. This preliminary preparation of materials and parts for arranged projects will lead to slightly more complicated operations, which will be more suited to Grade II patients, while the more complex work will be reserved for Grade III patients. It will be noted, therefore, that even individual projects in woodcraft will provide a wide range of treatment services for all grades of patients and the simultaneous arrangement of many widely differing projects will create treatment facilities for a vast number of patients involving many differing mental conditions. This capacity to provide occupation for large numbers, simultaneously, renders woodworking one of the most highly adaptable of the crafts used for therapeutic purposes.

(c) *Flexibility:* The wide and graduated range of complexity, as well as the high degree of adaptability present in woodworking, renders it also one of the most flexible of the therapeutic crafts. This flexibility is, in addition, enhanced by the absence of restriction in regard to location, as the various operations associated with all forms of timbercraft will embrace activities not exclusively confined to the workshop. The wide range of operations create novelty and variety, which render this craftwork one of the most popular and attractive of the occupations. This is borne out by the large number of widely differing and interesting articles that may be produced under therapeutic conditions. It is difficult to make an exclusive list, but the following will exemplify the point:—

(1) *Wooden Toys:* These are of such an extensive range that it is almost impossible to give a complete list of articles and the element of originality may be reflected in the ingenuity displayed in producing novel and exclusive designs. They might be classified into (a) *Simple,* (b) *Mechanical* and (c) *Elaborate.* (a) The *simple* range of toys would be exemplified by small wooden animals, building blocks, miniature wagons, motor lorries, boxes, sand spades, etc. (b) *Mechanical* toys would cover all the various simple miniature wheeled toys, such as small wheelbarrows, wagons, motor lorries, simply-constructed trams, engines, boats, animal shapes on wheels, etc. (c) *Elaborate* wooden toys would embrace close replicas, mainly in miniature, of various transport and other articles, as detailed under (b) *mechanical,* but involving additional and more elaborate details with regard to both mechanism and finish. Elaborately constructed dolls' houses and large rocking-horses might be included under this head.

(2) *Furniture Manufacture* comprises the production of a large range of articles, embracing great variety in design

and construction. These consist of chairs, couches, tables, cabinets, side-boards, kitchen furniture, bedroom furniture, bookcases, stools, firescreen frames, bookshelves and special items, such as folding and other card tables, tea or dinner trolleys, dumb-waiters, trays, etc. Practically all the items listed may be produced in a range of designs, involving many different shapes and operational techniques. This almost never-ending variety in construction and design creates an inimitable degree of novelty, which gives to woodworking its exceptionally high rating in flexibility and consequent therapeutic value.

(3) *Carpentry* or general construction covers a wide extent of timberwork in the manufacture of architectural and general requirements. This would include making doors, windows, partitions and other such items of house construction, as well as many articles required for outdoor use. These latter would include farm and garden, as well as other external requirements, such as gates, posts, railings, fences, wheelbarrows, carts, handbarrows, boxes of all kinds and shapes, workshop appliances, such as woodworking benches, toolchests, grindstone frames, etc., also such garden accessories as bee-hives, poultry houses, greenhouses, garden frames, summerhouses, etc.

(4) *Carving:* This is a specialised form of woodworking, with special tools and techniques, which may provide therapeutic occupation for a limited number of patients. The work is capable of being graded from rather simple complex to a high stage of complexity. It is only the simpler type of work that is of therapeutic interest and this must have obvious limitations. The general appearance of articles in wood may be substantially enhanced by the introduction of simple carving effects in some of the parts. The special tools consist of a variety of chisels and gauges, both straight and curved, as well as fluted, also some grounding and bordering punches.

(5) *Fretwork* or *Scroll Sawing* is a type of woodworking of therapeutic value, as it does not embrace very skilled or complicated operations and involves few tools. These consist merely of fretsaws and a small drill to provide the opening hole for the fretwork. The fretsaws may be of the

hand type or mechanical type worked by an electric motor. There is a semi-mechanical type worked by treadle, which increases its therapeutic value, by the additional introduction of footwork to operate the saw. All fretsaws, including the hand type, provide for the use of different grades of saw blades from the very finest to the coarsest. The finishing of the fret cuts will necessitate a round file and some sand-paper. The monotony of fretcutting is offset by the almost endless range of designs that are available. These may be used as a *gallery* for the tops of cabinets and other items of furniture, or as *stretchers* to provide ornamentation on many articles, such as tables, etc.

(6) *Repairs:* In all hospitals, particularly the large types, there is continuous occupation provided in dealing with woodwork repairs. All movable articles, such as furniture and other such items, may be dealt with as a special section in the woodcraft centre, while a mobile unit may be arranged to attend to wood repairs *in situ*, such as floors, windows, doors, etc.

(7) *Whittling* may be described as a hobby in woodcraft, consisting of the simple carving of small timber pieces into fancy articles, by the sole use of a sharpened penknife. Its limited therapeutic value is based more on recreation than handicraft grounds because of its diversional rather than utilitarian motivating force. Viewed as a hobby or otherwise, it does provide therapeutic occupation when prescribed.

(d) *Utility:* The serviceability of timbercraft in relation to hospital requirements places it at the head of all other therapeutic occupations. The ever-recurring repair work in wood, as well as the provision of timber articles, whether by replacement or addition, create a very beneficial arrangement of services for the hospital, whose treatment value is in no way lessened thereby. The combining of the utilitarian with the therapeutic element is effected in this craft as in no other and with mutual benefit.

### 2—*Economic*

In woodworking, the economic, as distinct from the therapeutic considerations, require analysis for comparative purposes. These are discussed under the following three heads:—(A) *Materials*, (B) *Equipment* and (C) *Disposal of Products*.

(A) *The materials* required for woodworking consist mainly of the various timbers suitable for craftwork, as well as a number of ancillary articles, such as glue, nails, screws, hinges, locks and other metal and plastic fitments, etc.

The raw material in wood consists of seasoned cuttings from different types of trees in various sizes and shapes to requirements. In this respect, it may be possible to organise associated occupations in tree-felling, log-cutting and subsequent seasoning, etc. The type of wood to be used will be dependent on the nature of the proposed project. There are well over one hundred different types of woods, but, in general use, these are reduced mainly to white deal, red deal, oak, mahogany, ash, beech, birch, pine (white or red), walnut and larch.

In addition to the latter timbers, special, additional woods are used for carving, cabinet-making, toy-making, etc. For carving, the following woods are mainly used: oak, mahogany, lime, pear, cherry, sycamore, yew, holly and chestnut.

For *Fretwork*, birch or oak plywoods are much in demand and easily worked. Maple, of the bird's eye type, black walnut, white holly, Spanish cedar and rosewood are also used.

In *Toy-making* the timber used must be light and consists generally of white deal, white and red pine, white canary-wood. Spruce and larch are also used, when available. The playing pieces for chess and draughts are made from such woods as holly, lime, birch and sycamore, while the more expensive types are made of boxwood, ebony or lignum vitae.

In *Turnery* the woods generally used are birch, ash or beech, while finials are turned in boxwood or similar hardwoods. Satinwood is also used, in particular, for backing hair-brushes and clothes-brushes, etc.

In *Cabinet-making* and furniture manufacture, a variety of woods is also used, the more usual being oak, maple, mahogany, walnut, rose, teak, cherry, pear, plane and birch (the cherry type known as *mahogany birch*). Cheaper types of cabinets and furniture are made from white deal, lime and the pines, the latter forming the groundwork for most veneer-work. For special cabinet inlaying, the Killarney arbutus, yew (*Taxis Hibernicus*) and holly give a very beautiful finish and effect. For special fancy articles of furniture, including particularly pianos, as well as veneering, the Tasmanian muskwood is often used.

For special purposes, persimmon is used for shuttle-making, golfclub heads and wood-engraving. Pear wood, apart from furniture, is also used for making cog-wheels, rollers and screws for wine-presses.

Willow is used for making handles of cricket bats and other such equipment, as well as toys. The Palm willow, because of its toughness and elasticity, is used for tool handles. Ash, birch and beech are also turned for handles of tools, while the former is used for the manufacture of hurling and hockey sticks and other similar items of sporting equipment.

Hickory or white walnut, because of its elasticity and toughness, is used for fishing-rods, handles for tools, gun-stocks, the shafts of horse carriages, etc. In cases where weight is a special consideration, such as trays, etc., the Lombardy Poplar (*Populus Dilatata*) is much used, as it is the lightest of the several species of poplar, all of which are characterised by their lightness and durability, with little tendency to shrink or swell. Poplar, because of its softness and absence of splitting, is a good carving wood. It is also used in the manufacture of paper.

For the production of articles or for use in situations where contact with water is an important consideration, there is no wood to excel the well-known Eastern Teak (*Tectoma Grandis*). It has the additional advantages of being very strong, though light and easily worked. Because of these special qualities, teak is one of the leading woods used in ship-building and likewise is the principal wood used for drainers in kitchen or scullery sinks, etc.

This incomplete listing of the many woods used for constructive purposes of all kinds demonstrates the wide variety of choice available for O.T. activities. Considerations, however, additional to those of purpose and cost, must enter into the choice of material for all woodworking projects. Facility for easy working, because of softness and lightness, is an important consideration. In this respect, lime and walnut, at different ends of the economic pole, claim first attention. They also are of light weight, which is another strong recommendation in their favour and they will meet the needs of most O.T. woodworking projects. For a host of general purpose requirements, deal and, in particular, the white variety, if chosen as free from knots as possible, stands out as the chief raw material of all O.T. departments.

Mention must also be made of oak as an important general purpose material. Its ubiquitous quality strengthens its claim for recognition, as it grows in practically every country in Europe, as well as in different parts of America, Canada, Africa, Asia, Australia and India. Oak, however, has the disadvantage of being rather heavy for working, particularly the West African and *durmast* type (*Quercus Pubescens*). The most highly recommended oak for craft purposes is the *Wainscot* type, found mainly in Holland and Riga, because it is soft and, consequently, easy to work and does not tend to split or warp. In addition, it possesses the well known silver grain, which enhances its value for appearance and finish.

The unlimited world supply of raw materials for woodworking, even when limited to native sources arising from the restrictive effects of world war or similar conditions, gives the craft an advantage probably unequalled by any other in this respect. The effects of global wars in cutting off the supply of raw materials for most handicrafts, which reduces the extent of normal O.T. services, while it may restrict the extent of woodworking projects, does not lead to suspension of this craft. The large variety of timbers, native in all countries, provides ample substitutes to permit continuation of the craft for treatment purposes.

In addition, woodworking possesses an unique advantage in having available in all large hospitals a wealth of waste material, readily convertible into myriads of useful products at practically no cost. Waste pieces of timber, as well as discarded boxes and packing cases and excess material following repair projects, create an almost continuous supply of materials to operate a special treatment unit in most hospitals.

(B) *Equipment*, apart from the (1) *special carpenter's bench* and such accessories as nails, screws, etc., consists mainly of (2) the *various Tools* required for the many different operations associated with woodworking of all kinds.

(1) *The Bench* may be purchased or, better still, made in the woodworking centre. The size of the bench varies from 6 feet to 4 feet in length, 2 feet to $1\frac{1}{2}$ feet in width and $2\frac{3}{4}$ feet to $2\frac{1}{2}$ feet in height in accordance with requirements. The best type is made of beech, but a satisfactory and very serviceable one can be constructed in good quality white deal. It must be of a strong, rigid type to withstand planing and sawing, with an even and smooth surface. Some of the commercial types on offer are of a portable pattern, consisting of steel frame legs, easily dismantled or assembled by means of iron screw bolts, which give the bench a necessary rigidity. The wooden top may be of white deal or beech and is supplied with a number of useful fitments, such as a quickly adjusting grip vice, screw rising stop, a nest of drawers, as well as a bench-knife, fitting into different pegged positions on the bench, to suit the differing lengths of boards to be worked. The bench-knife has an adjustable arm, operated by a small lever and cam, which keeps the work rigid between itself and the bench-stop. The bench should be fixed in the optimum position with regard to light and floor space. This is generally against the wall of the workshop immediately underneath a window, so that the light plays on the work.

(2) *Tools* may be classified as follows: (a) *Rasping*, (b) *Edge*, (c) *Striking*, (d) *Boring*, (e) *Chopping*, (f) *Grinding* and (g) *Holding*.

(a) *Rasping tools* consist of the many different types of saws, as well as rasps and files. *Saws* are tools used for cutting and dividing materials, mainly wood, and consist of a thin plate of steel with sharp teeth on the cutting edge.

*Saws* are mainly divided into *Handsaws* and *Machine*

*Saws* and the former again into *those with* and *those without Backs*. *Saws with Backs* are of four kinds: *Tenon, Sash, Dovetail* and *Carcass*. *Saws without Backs* are classified as follows: *Handsaws, Rip-saws, Panel-saws, Table-saws, Siding-saws, Keyhole-saws* and *Lock-saws*.

*Machine saws* are of three types: (1) *Circular*, (2) *Jig-saws*, also known as *Fret* or *Reciprocating saws* and (3) *Band-saws*. *Circular saws* are available in many different sizes, from the small bench type, suitable for O.T. departments, to the large powerful types used for tipping and cross-cutting huge tree logs.

*Files* and *Rasps* are pieces of steel from 12 to 24 inches in length, generally flat, though they may be triangular-shaped, with grooved or toothed surfaces, suitable for smoothing or sanding down wood, leather, iron and such substances. Files differ from rasps in having single or crossed diagonally placed straight furrows, while rasps have single teeth, which have been punched up to give a coarser effect on the surface to be treated. Files vary in fineness to give either a double cut or a float cut. Rasps vary also in size of teeth to give coarser or finer results as required, ranging from the large-toothed horse type to the much smaller-toothed smooth type.

(b) *Edge-Tools* include a number of special cutting tools, comprising *Planes, Chisels, Gouges, Spokeshaves*, as well as sharpening tools, such as *Oilstones, Grindstones*, etc.

*Chisels* differ from *Gouges* in that the former have a straight cutting edge, while the latter are more or less curved. *Chisels* are either of the morticing or paring type; the former ranging from $\frac{1}{8}$ inch to 1 inch in cutting width, increasing by 1/16th inch at a time, while the latter extend from $\frac{1}{8}$ inch to 2 inches in width, increasing by $\frac{1}{8}$ inch at a time. *Gouges* have a similar range to paring chisels in each of 8 different degrees of curve. The curvature in the gouges ranges from very flat to a deep half-circle type, known as fluting. The eight curves in question are known as very flat, flat, two degrees of middle curve, two degrees of scribing curve, half fluting and fluting—all eight degrees available in each of the different widths noted above.

The *Spokeshave* may be described as an ordinary razor type of knife embedded on one side of a handle, bearing a hand-grip at each end and used for cutting on the safety-razor principle, the action being similar to, but the reverse of, that of the plane. It differs from the plane in that the depth of shave cut with each motion is not adjustable as in the case of the plane. It has the advantage over the plane of being more efficient where the surface to be dealt with is very curved and grossly uneven. The more usual long-bladed type of spokeshave is also available in cutters of different forms for purposes of rabbeting or chamfering, etc., described in the U.S.A. as *routers*.

The *Plane* consists of a type of adjustable chisel, inserted into a solid wooden block of wood (also of metal), with the cutting edge projecting at an angle through the smooth-faced bottom of the block. There are three general types of planes in use, known as (1) *the Jack-plane*, (2) *the Trying-plane* and (3) *the Smoothing-plane*. All three are more or less alike, differing in general only in size and in certain characteristics special to each, which lead also to functional differences. Timber received from the sawmills requires to be smoothed and rendered true and straight for constructional purposes. This levelling and smoothing is effected by the three types of planes—the initial trueing being carried out by the *Jack-plane*, improved on by the *Trying-plane* and finally completed by the *Smoothing-plane*. The *Jack-plane* and *Trying-plane* are only differentiated by the shorter length of the former, about 15 inches as against 18 to 24 inches and the variation in the shape of the handle. The iron of the *Jack-plane* is also narrower than that of the *Trying-plane* and has a convex cutting edge in comparison with the straight edge of the latter. The iron of the *Smoothing-plane* is somewhat similar to that of the *Trying-plane* and, as its name suggests, is used for smoothing off any irregularities of surface left after the *Jack-plane*. There are special planes also used, known as *Rabbet* or *Rebate-planes* and *Plough-planes*. These are used for cutting rebates or recesses in surfaces, where required.

(c) *Striking Tools* consist of the familiar *hammers* and

*mallets* so essential in woodworking. *Hammers* are of various sizes and shapes and of various weights, ranging from ½ ounce to 10 lbs. and heavier. For woodworking purposes they are of two types; the *plain Exeter type*, which is used for striking solely and the *Claw-hammer*, which has an additional claw attachment to facilitate drawing nails, etc.

*Mallets* are simply hammers, with a wooden instead of steel head and are of the square-headed or round-headed type. They are generally used for chiselling or for use on wooden surfaces that would otherwise be damaged if struck with a steel hammer.

(d) *Boring Tools* consist of *Bits* and *Braces*, *Gimlets*, *Augers*, *Awls* and *Drills*, and are used for boring holes of different sizes for various purposes. The *awl* or *bradawl* is the simplest of these tools and consists of a steel rod attached to a timber handle with the other end of the rod doubly bevelled to a sharp edge. It produces the hole by displacement of the wood fibres, without cutting or removing them. The speed and efficiency of the bradawl, in preparing soft woods to take a nail or screw, cannot be equalled as a hand tool. It is, however, not so suitable in the case of hardwoods. *Gimlets* are adaptations of the *awl* with a screw-point and generally with a T-shaped handle to facilitate the screwing motion in its operation. Subsequent development of the *gimlet* led to the introduction of the *auger*, which is simply an enlarged type of *gimlet* where the two hands are used for the screwing operation and with a twisted or spiral type of shank. The *gimlet* and, to some extent, the *auger* have been replaced by the *brace and bit* and the *drill*. The latter two are somewhat similar, in that they obviate the interrupted motion of the hands as when using the *gimlet* or *auger*. The *simple type of brace* consists of a simple crank, one end of which has a round head to allow the workman to exert pressure on the tool with his breast, while the other end has an adaptable recess for the insertion of the auger-like bits of varying sizes and shapes. The centre of the crank has a grip-shaped arrangement to enable the brace to be turned by the hand, with a horizontal circular motion. The bits are usually held in the lower end of the crank by means of a thumb-screw, which grips into the notch so provided, in the stem-end of each bit. The *drill* is of the bit and brace type, where the crank is replaced with a straight shaft to the side of which is attached a hand-operated gear wheel which rotates the lower end of the shaft or chuck. This chuck has a similar arrangement to that of the brace for holding the different-sized bits. The gear wheel on the side of the shaft is operated by the hand in a vertical manner, which gives easier and more efficient working.

(e) *Chopping Tools* refer to *Edge-Tools*, which are used with a striking motion and, consequently, have a much stronger cutting edge than the latter. They consist of a steel head with a cutting edge attached to the familiar type of curved timber handle and are of three kinds: *Hatchets*, *Axes* and *Adzes*.

*Hatchets* and *Axes* are similar in structure, except that hatchets are much smaller and for single-handed use. Axes, requiring the use of both hands, have a longer handle attached to a heavier and thicker head with a narrow or broad cutting edge, as required. The cutting edge in all cases is of the bevelled, convex type. The *Adze* may be described as an axe with a curved blade in the head, which facilitates the cutting of a concave surface and is generally so used by wheelwrights in the hand-manufacture of felloes or curved rims of timber wheels. The special technique required for the operation of an adze, as well as a certain risk in its use, does not make it a suitable tool for O.T. craftwork.

(f) *Guiding Tools* consist of *Hand-rules*, *Squares*, *Straight-edges*, *Levels*, *Gauges*, *Mitre-boxes*, *Bevels*, *Compasses* and *Calipers*, *Trammels*, etc., usually seen among the many different items of the woodworker's equipment. The familiar *Foot-rule* needs no description and is one of the most essential of all O.T. tools for a variety of purposes. *Squares* are most useful tools for accurately marking work at right angles and generally consist of a wooden stock with a steel blade riveted or screwed on at right angles. They are of various sizes to suit small or large work and a T-shaped one, known as a *mitre square*, is also used.

The *Straight-edge*, as the name suggests, is merely a long piece of planed board (also available in steel) varying in length from 6 feet to 12 feet or more and about 4 to 6 inches in width, in accordance with its length, with the two long edges perfectly straight and parallel to each other. It is used for testing the evenness of a surface by laying it on top of the surface to be tested. It is also used in conjunction with the spirit level, for testing horizontal or ground levels.

*Levels* are mainly of two kinds: *Spirit Levels* and *Plumb Levels*. The latter, generally used by masons, are for gauging true perpendicularity of constructional work, whether of timber or otherwise. They consist of a straight edge with a small weight suspended from the centre of the top end of the straight edge by a cord. When the cord coincides with a fixed line marked down the exact centre of the wide part of the straight edge, when laid upright beside the work to be tested, it indicates that the latter is in true perpendicular. The *Spirit Level*, though generally used to indicate when work is truly horizontal, may also be used as a plumb level, when it possesses an additional tube of spirit laid in a circular opening, close to one end of the level at right angles to the main tube of spirit, which is encased flush with the main upper surface of the block of the level. Each of the two tubes in question are incompletely filled with spirit so that, when either tube of the level is placed in the horizontal position, a bubble of air appears in the middle of the tube and each tube is accordingly adjusted in place in the block of the level, so that the bubble appears in the marked centre of a sight-hole in a metallic plate covering each tube, thus indicating that the level is in the truly horizontal or truly vertical position respectively.

*Gauges* are of three kinds, described respectively as the *marking*, the *cutting* and the *mortice gauge*. The first two differ only in that the *marking gauge* has a single, fixed spike, with an adjustable, sliding head, common to both, while the *cutting gauge* has a small steel plate, sharpened on one edge, so as to make a cut in the work, generally for dovetailing. The *mortice gauge* is of the same structure as the marking and cutting gauges, except that it has two marking spikes instead of one. One of these spikes is fixed and the other is capable of being adjusted at varying distances from the fixed one, so as to give a double gauging to facilitate making mortices and tenons.

The *Mitre-box* is a narrow box-shaped rectangular structure with saw-cuts made at half a right angle across the two sides of the box to facilitate the accurate cutting of work by guiding the saw at this angle over the timber to be cut, when inserted in the box. Its use is illustrated best in the angular cuts made in picture framing to ensure accurate joining at the four corners of the frame assembly.

The *Bevel* may be simply described as a type of adjustable square for marking work at every degree of angle, additional to that of right angle. They are made of wood or steel and may be of the ordinary hinged type or of the hinged type with a sliding arrangement for the bevel.

*Compasses* and *Calipers* have a double function. They are generally used for marking off circular figures where required, but are also used for gauging dimensions, where a rule cannot be used. They are usually made of steel of varying sizes and designs to suit requirements. The *Trammel* may be described as a type of compass, used for striking very large circles. They are not made, like the compass, with the two sharply pointed legs hinged together at the other end. The pointed legs are attached to a bar, on which they slide to provide markings at adjustable lengths and used in the manner of the compass above. One of the adjustable legs may be provided with a thumb-screw arrangement for attaching a lead pencil.

(g) *Holding Tools* consist of *Vices*, *Pincers* and *Clamps* or *Cramps*.

*Vices* are either of the *hand* or *bench type*. *Hand Vices* are of many patterns, including the simple hinged-type with adjustable screw for the jaws, a sliding jaw type on a fixed handle and a ball and socket type for saw filing. The adjustable chuck of a brace or drill is an example of a pin vice. The *Bench Vice*, which is attached to the carpenter's bench, is available in several different types of design, the most popular being that with a sliding arrangement of the jaws, which enables them to be closed or drawn in one single movement. *Clamps* are used for closing up the joints in boards, whether for nailing or to ensure hardening in glue-work. *A special G-Cramp* is used for holding picture frames together after glueing and can be procured with a ball and socket arrangement for holding work together, which is not square. There is also a *corner type of Clamp* for holding together the two mitred ends of a picture frame at a perfect right angle, while nailing, screwing or glueing together. *Pincers* and *Pliers* do not require description, either as to design or function. They are made in various sizes and qualities to suit different requirements.

(C) *Disposal of Products:* The universal demand for wood products, apart from the question of repairs and maintenance, simplifies the problem of disposal. This is particularly so in the mental hospital, where the constant demand for articles and replacements in wood, as well as internal and external repairs, is often more than sufficient to maintain one form of a continuous treatment service. It may be necessary, in fact, from time to time, to expand the activities of the woodworking section to cover the manifold hospital needs in wooden products of all kinds.

In addition, there is often a request for the supply of an article in wood to a special design, which is not available from normal market sources. This obviates the disposal problem, as here the demand creates production rather than production seeking subsequent outlet. Further, the possibility of producing a wide range of wooden toys, both of the large and small type, which, when subsequently finished in a host of bright, attractive colours, make their disposal a simple matter during pre-'Xmas trade demands.

# CHAPTER XVI.

## SPECIAL CRAFT ANALYSIS

### WOODCRAFT (*contd.*)

#### 3—*Technical*

THE TECHNICAL side in woodcraft reveals a medley of operations, which follow naturally from the many and varied tools already described, as well as from the many different types of wood used and the multiplicity of products resulting therefrom. The list of projects that are undertaken in manufactures, made up mainly in wooden materials, creates almost as many operations as essential tools. A classification of these may, accordingly, be based on that already outlined for the various tools, as follows: (A) *Cutting* associated with saws, (B) *Planing* and *Paring* connected with the various types of edge-tools, (C) *Striking Operations* involving hammers and mallets. (D) *Boring* work as carried out with the different drills, augers, gimlets, etc. (E) *Chopping* operations connected with the use of axes, hatchets and adzes. (F) *Guiding Activities* associated with the different levels, bevels, rules, etc., and (G) *Holding Operations* connected with vices, clamps, etc. It must be appreciated, however, that all these operations are definitely inter-related and many of them are in close association in carrying out any individual project. Thus, cutting, planing and paring are facilitated by the use of both guiding and holding tools. Boring operations are also of preliminary use in cutting out circular pieces, as well as in morticing, etc.

(A) *Cutting* is generally the first and most important operation in dealing with prepared timber, which is carried out by the use of suitable saws and varies with the kind of saw used, whether that of the hand or machine type. Sawing is of two main kinds: (1) *coarse* or *preparatory* and (2) *fine* or *adaptive*.

(1) The initial *coarse sawing* is carried out in the conversion of logs into suitable planks or boards by means of large,

ripping type of power-operated circular saws. Additional preparatory cutting of these planks and boards may be carried out in the main woodworking section of the O.T. department, by either small bench circular saws or by the coarser type of handsaws, which are represented by those without backs.

The movements involved in machine cutting, apart from preliminary lifting, consist mainly in gripping and gently pushing with the hands. In handwork with single-grip saws, the chief movements, all one-handed, are alternate flexion and extension of the elbow with mild circumduction of the shoulder joint of a short lateral type. All these movements are of a continuous, repetitive nature during the actual sawing operations. There is, in addition, a continuous gripping with a fixed flexion of the finger joints of both hands. In hand cross-cut saws, operated by two persons, the latter flexion is confined mainly to one hand and the extension movement of the elbow has a strongly passive element during the active elbow flexion by the other operator.

(2) *The fine or adaptive* type of sawing may be of the hand or machine type. The latter is carried out by small, bench, circular, fine-toothed saws, which are used in all well-equipped O.T. departments. Jig or reciprocating saws, used generally for fretwork, perform cutting of a fine type. The movements associated with these machines are somewhat similar to the grosser type of circular saws described, but a higher degree of concentration is required in the finer type of sawing.

The movements involved in using the smaller backless saws, including tenon saws, are more or less similar to those associated with the larger saws described above, except that they are more reduced in amplitude and less energy-expending. They would, accordingly, be more suitable as remedial exercises for conditions associated with the joints concerned in the earlier and more acute stages.

(B) *Planing and Paring* may be described as specialised cutting operations carried out with the various edge tools, comprising planes, chisels, gouges, spokeshaves, etc. While sawing has a preparatory function in reducing large work to more suitable working sizes, it has, also, in common with planing, the special purpose of adapting the latter to the actual and final proportions required for project construction. *Planing*, likewise, has an additional function in creating flat, smooth surfaces in the constructional parts, where required. *Planing*, as the name implies, is associated, exclusively, with the different types of planes, while paring is carried out by means of chisels, spokeshaves and gouges. The latter are used for a special form of paring in the formation of grooves, etc.

Timber, requiring to be planed, is laid flat on the bench, one end against a special *stop* to immobilise the wood, while the plane is moved along in the direction of the grain. In a Jack-plane, the handle is gripped generally by the right hand, with the forefinger extended towards the centre wedge, while the left hand grips the front portion of the stock, with the thumb placed on the near side of the plane. The Trying-plane is gripped in a similar manner, but differs in that the pressure of the arms does not remain uniform throughout each stroke, as with the Jack-plane. With the Trying-plane there is increased pressure of the left arm during the first half of the stroke and of the right arm for the last half. The Smoothing-plane, in the absence of a handle, is held by the right hand gripping immediately behind the knife, while the left hand grasps the front end with the thumb pressing on the top of the stock. The rabbeting plane is gripped in a somewhat similar manner to that of the latter.

The movements involved in planing are, in the main, similar to those associated with the finer types of hand-sawing, with the variations in gripping, etc. already noted. The joint movements involved, likewise, vary in amplitude according to the size of the plane used.

*Paring* is carried out generally with the different types of chisels and, to a lesser extent, by means of the spokeshave. In the light or finer work, this is done by holding the chisel in the right hand while the wood is held tightly by the left hand, but well behind the tool to obviate accidents. The chisel is operated with a thrusting motion, taking precaution that the tool edge does not come in additional contact with anything of a hard nature that might damage it, such as the rough surface of the bench, etc. The grip of the right hand on the chisel varies as between vertical and horizontal paring. In the latter, the forefinger is extended along the handle, while, in the former, the handle is gripped with all fingers in dagger-like fashion.

In cutting *mortices* and *tenons*, a mallet is used to strike the chisel, which is held securely in the left hand. Care must be taken to hold the chisel at a suitable angle to prevent what is described as 'undercutting' or achieving the opposite effect. This can be avoided in making a mortice, by cutting it from both sides to half-way in each case. This method will facilitate the finishing-off of the mortice at the correct angle and thus secure a close-fitting joint by avoiding any 'undercutting' of the hole. While a blunt chisel may be used in the initial stages of the work, care must be taken to prevent bruising of the wood fibres, particularly in soft woods, by using a keenly-sharpened chisel for finishing the sides of the mortice.

Gouges are held in the same way as a paring chisel, but, when used with the mallet, should always be held perpendicularly.

Spokeshaves are not in general use in O.T. departments, but they are useful tools to substitute for planes or chisels, when dealing with round curved work. They are worked in both directions, from and towards the operator. As they are gripped with both hands, the movements result in simultaneous, alternating extension and flexion of both elbow joints, with some flexion of the wrist joints.

(C) *Striking Operations:* The use of hammers and mallets, particularly the former, is commonplace in all O.T. departments, even apart from woodworking. No special technical knowledge is required for their operation. Extension of the right elbow, followed by flexion, are the main movements involved, with the greater emphasis on extension. The amplitude of the movements concerned will, of course, depend on the size and weight of the hammer used. In the heavier types of hammering, where both hands are used, as in the case of sledges, in addition to the muscles of both arms, those in the lumbar region and to a much lesser extent the leg muscles, are also brought into play.

(D) *Boring Work:* The use of awls, drills and such tools introduce an element of variety which is such a notable feature of woodworking of all kinds. In hand boring, the chief movements are connected with the wrist and finger joints of the right hand, with some flexion and alternating pronation and supination. The left hand grips the wood being worked. In the case of the bit and brace, as well as the hand drill, there is limited flexion of the right elbow joints. The auger, also, being a two-handed tool, has similar limited flexion, but of both elbow joints alternately and what is characteristically more important, there is pronation and supination of both wrists of a rhythmic, alternating character.

(E) *Chopping Operations:* The use of hatchets, axes and adzes, confined, as they are, to the grosser and less technical operations in woodworking, may be regarded as a special, though more or less identical operation to that of striking. Like hammers, the extent and amplitude of the movements involved depend on the weight and size of the tool used. Axes require greater effort, with greater extent of movement, than those associated with hatchets. Adzes, however, requiring more skill in control and greater dexterity in use, have a very limited application, if any, in O.T. craftwork.

(F) *Guiding and Holding Activities:* As these activities deal, merely, with the use of ancillary tools, such as rules, levels, bevels, vices, etc., they do not call for any technical discussion in the woodworking activities of the O.T. department and are similarly used in other types of craftwork.

## Special Technical Operations

Constructional work with wood involves specialised operations, varying in technical grade and may be classified under the two main heads of (i) *Jointwork* and (ii) *Fastening.*

### i—Jointwork

There is a large variety of joints to deal with in the many constructional problems associated with woodworking and these have been listed as follows: (a) Those dealing with the *Lengthening* of beams, such as *lapping, fishing, scarfing, tabling* and *building-up:* (b) Those for *Bearing*, such as *halving, notching, dovetailing, cogging, housing, tusk-tenoning* and *chase-morticing* and (c) *Miscellaneous Joints*, such as *mortice and tenon, mitre, rabbet (rebate) and butt-joints.*

(a) *Lapping* is the simplest method of jointing for the lengthening of two beams. The overlapped portions of the two beams being held together by steel strap surrounds or by through-bolts, with oak or steel keys inserted between and into beams to prevent sliding in the joint. In the simple type of *fishing* joint, the beam ends butt against each other, with timber or steel straps above and below the joint held in position by through-bolts, with or without intervening keys. A joint is described as *scarfed* or *tabled* when portions of the ends of the beams are bedded into each other longitudinally. This type of joint is not in common use and many different types of scarfing are described, dependent on the shape of the scarf, whether it is cut square and parallel or with an incline. The scarf may also be of the tongued variety and may be held with wedges and may be of the vertical or longitudinal type. The difference between the scarfed and finished type of joint is merely that, in the latter, there is no shortening of the beams, as they are butted against each other and there is no overlapping as in the former. A *building-up* type of joint consists in laying two or more beams sideways and bolting them together, generally with or without a wrought-iron plate between. When several pieces are so bolted together, an increased shortening effect is produced by keeping the individual fished joints in different positions in the bolted section.

(b) *Bearing* joints are so called because the beams concerned carry a load across the grain. The simplest type of bearing joint is the *halving-joint* where two pieces of cross bracing are halved together, leaving the cross pieces flush with each other on top and bottom of the joint. In a *notching* joint, the cross pieces are not flush with each other and may be of the single or double-notched type, according as the notch is made in only one of the cross pieces or in both. A bearing-joint of the *dovetailed* variety is merely a halving joint, where the cut of the intersection is made at a slight angle to the horizontal plane of the beams, giving a bevelled appearance. A *cogging* joint is a notched joint where the notch in the lower beam is incompletely cut, leaving a cog of timber, uncut, across the middle of the notch. A *housing joint* is a type of tenon joint, where one piece of wood is let bodily into a mortice in another for a short distance. This is commonly used in stair-cases and also for fixing rails to uprights for fencing purposes. *Tusk-tenoning* is used to secure a bearing for a beam meeting another at right angles on the same level. It is used for fireplace surrounds and similar openings in floors and has the advantage of securing a good bearing, without substantially weakening the beam. *Chase-morticing* is used to attach a cross beam into two beams already fixed in position. The mortice made in each of the latter is chased out in a horizontal direction, but in opposite directions, to permit the cross piece, with reverse tenons, to slide into their respective mortices.

(c) Of the *Miscellaneous Joints* listed, that of the simple *tenon and mortice* type is the more generally used, whether fixed with wedges or dowels (pins). There are as many types of tenons available for construction as there are varieties in shape and many of them have been given special names, such as the *tusk*, *dovetailed* and *housing* types already described. A *fox-tail* tenon, of dovetailed shape, is used for joining small pieces, but is difficult to fix and not much used. A *joggle* tenon is a stub-shaped piece on the top of an upright or sill to which a cross beam is attached to prevent the latter getting out of position. Tenons may also be of the double-pronged type for use in attaching wide frame pieces.

## ii—*Fastenings*

In addition to the various joints described, there are ancillary as well as additional methods of fastening in timber construction, such as: (a) *Wedges*, (b) *Pins*, (c) *Keys*, (d) *Sockets*, (e) *Straps*, (f) *Glue* and (g) *Hinging*.

(a) *Wedges* consist of timber pieces usually split or torn off from their original part, to ensure continuity of the grain. They are often, however, cut by saw from straight-grained pieces and must just have enough taper to give proper compression in the joint where used. If used for external purposes, they should be coated with white lead before use, as this is more resistant than glue to moisture.

(b) *Pins* for wood fastening are made of wood or steel. The latter include nails, screws, bolts and spikes. Wooden pins, like wedges, are made from hard, straight-grained woods. They are generally round in shape, though square pins are more efficient though rarely used, owing to the difficulty of making accurate square holes. Used mainly to make tenons secure in mortices, the round pins are known as dowels. They are also used to secure flooring boards together, though the tongued and grooved method of flooring is of more universal use.

Nails are either of the cut or wrought iron type. Cut nails, which are available in a multiplicity of sizes, are used to a very large extent in wood construction for general purposes. For special purposes, particularly where dismantling may be necessary, *steel screws* are used. Wooden nails are known as *treenails* and are often used to secure railway chairs to sleepers. The fact that they swell when exposed to moisture, tends to increase their holding power. *Spikes* are merely nails of the giant type and are used only for heavy timber construction. *Bolts* are also used in heavy constructional work and always with washers both at the head as well as the butt end, to prevent too much penetration of the wood on securely tightening.

(c) *Keys* are small strips of wood or metal inserted into adjoining pieces of wood to keep them in position. They may be of the *internal* or *external* type, according as they are used in between two pieces or beams lying parallel together or when inserted across a right-angled dovetailed joint, as at the angle formed by two sides of a box. The latter may be a metal strip, corrugated in shape, driven into the joint or it may be a thin strip of glued wood inserted into a saw cut made across the joint.

(d) *Sockets* are cast iron boxes fixed into the ends of timber framing.

(e) *Straps* are iron bands placed across a joint to strengthen it. They are stirrup-shaped, when the strap is carried around a beam with both ends attached to the piece joining at right angles, as in the king-post sitting vertically on the horizontal tie-beam of a roof.

(f) *Glueing* is an important adjuvant in joint construction and does not require any technical elaboration in its use. It is recognised that the optimum results are achieved by using the best quality glue with the thinnest possible film.

(g) *Hinging* may be described simply as a form of movable joint, as when connecting two pieces of wood by means of a hinge, such as a door to the side of a frame, etc. Hinges are generally made of metal and of many different varieties, dependent on shape as well as purpose. Chief among them may be mentioned *butt, casement, garnet, desk, scuttle, chest, coach, rising, screw, centre-point, back-fold, H-hinges*, etc.

We have discussed the general, as well as some of the special technical operations associated with wood-working. It is not possible, however, with the obvious limitations of a textbook such as this, to treat in detail the manifold constructional projects that are possible under the general heading of woodworking. These varied activities will be embraced in a comprehensive manner in the practical or clinical side of the treatment, where they come within the immediate purview of the occupational therapist.

### 4—*Psychological*

The psychological considerations may be dealt with under two heads, namely: (a) *Nursing and Supervisory* and (b) *Mental processes involved*.

(a) *Nursing and supervisory responsibilities* are relatively increased in woodworking as compared with most other handicrafts and this is the only main disadvantage that tends to reduce the rating value of this occupation. The large variety of tools and machines available in the woodworking section, most of which are of the cutting type, necessitate active supervision of a more or less continuous nature. Patients with a melancholic symptomatology and, in particular, those suffering from suicidal tendencies, are very rarely submitted, under prescription, for general woodworking activities. This restricts its range of application for treatment purposes.

General experience, however, shows that the risks involved
are minimised, both by suitable prescription precautions
as well as the maintenance of adequate supervisory arrangements. The speedy modification of the more active symptoms
of melancholia and, in particular, the suicidal tendency,
through the influence of early Electro-Convulsant Therapy,
has opened up the craft as an auxiliary form of treatment in
suitable cases, that might, otherwise, have to be excluded
for the reasons stated.

(b) *The mental processes aroused* under the influence of woodworking in its many different phases of activity, may be
discussed under separate heads: (1) There is a heightening
of *interest* because of the novelty of the work and the wide
range of different activities, arising from the many and varied
tools brought into operation even in each single project.
Interest is, therefore, maintained in all stages of the work
and this counters any tendency to fatigue that might otherwise
arise from lack of emotional satisfaction and consequent
development of ennui. The persistent nature of the interest
aroused by a craft is the greatest possible single factor in
countering boredom, and there is probably no craft, where
stimulation of interest remains at such a high, continuous
level to the extent that it does in woodworking. It is, therefore, a highly stimulating occupation in its general activities,
though a sedative effect may be achieved through the repetitive operations occurring in part in individual projects.
(2) The amount of *concentration and attention* required in
woodworking activities may be regulated to suit the capacity
of the mental condition under treatment. This is readily
achieved because of the wide variety of projects and the many
different operations connected with the craft and, particularly,
as pointed out already, because this almost unending series
of projects and operations embraces all grades of complexity,
ranging from the very simplest type to the most complicated,
where maximum demands on attention and concentration
are called for. The discerning occupational therapist will
adapt these activities to meet the prescription requirements
in each individual case, making subsqeuent provision to
keep pace with the progress made or, if necessary, reducing

the complexity of the work to prevent the development of (3) *Fatigue*, arising from possible over-concentration of attention. This O.T. regulatory requirement has, in no other occupation, such a flexible basis as in the craft of wood-working. Fatigue, though occurring in this manner from psychological factors, is discussed in further detail in the following paragraphs.

### 5—*Physical*

Here the question of fatigue arises and its prevention is a *sine qua non* condition in the therapeutic development of this, as indeed of all forms of suitable craft work. This can be achieved, as already described, by (a) *suitable project selection*, (b) *proper working posture* and also by (c) *avoidance of other physical strains*, associated with the senses, such as *eye-strain*, etc. (a) The *nature of the project* must be gauged to conform with both the mental and physical capacities of each individual patient. The heavier type of projects require more muscular effort and is obviously unsuited for the patient of light physique or in those cases where the physical health is not at par. The multiplicity of projects, associated with all forms of woodworking, unequalled in this respect, facilitates suitable therapeutic selection. The wide range in complexity of the many operations and projects available in woodworking, provides for appropriate choice, in those cases where the element of fatigue is prone to rapid development, because of a lowered state of comprehension common to the acuter stages of most mental disorders.

(b) The question of *posture* in relation to the work under-taken is of vital importance in the prevention of fatigue. This is particularly so where the craft operation involves a more or less fixity of posture, which must lead to eventual fatigue. In woodworking, the vast bulk of the operations is carried out in the standing position, with constant and regular variations in body posture. This tends to reduce the possibility of posture fatigue. Some operations may allow of a sitting position and this affords a certain amount of relaxation, which may be necessary to interrupt the many long periods of standing that are not desirable in a large

percentage of psychotics. Here again the individual needs
in each case are paramount and the discerning occupational
therapist will adapt the project selection in accordance
with the prescription *designata* in each case.

(c) The most common factor in the development of *fatigue
arising from physical strain* associated with the bodily senses
is that due to *eye-strain*. The bulky nature of the materials
in general use in woodcraft projects tends to reduce
this to the very minimum and, consequently, does not call
for the same degree of attention as in other therapeutic
crafts. The varied nature of the operations that are often
associated in even one individual type of project is also a
factor in preventing eye-strain. In addition, the fact that the
optimum amount of light can be focussed on woodwork
activities, some being permissible in the outer daylight, is a
further preventive advantage. Some element of hearing-
strain may appear as a result of undue operational noises,
particularly when of the continuous type, such as those
associated with circular and other sawing activities,
hammering, etc. These objectionable sounds are rarely
of such a continuous nature as to prove of a serious therapeutic obstacle and, consequently, do not create any undue
restrictions in application.

### 6—*Advantages*

(A) From the points of view of *adaptability* and *flexibility*,
woodworking exhibits a very high rating in both respects.
There is a tremendous range of projects and operations
available in woodworking from the simplest to the most
complex, catering for all grades of patients and including
activities of both the sedative and stimulative type. This
marked element of adaptability raises the craft to an exceptionally high level in extent of application, almost on a par
with willowcraft and allied activities.

(B) From the *psychological standpoint*, (a) *the patient's
interest* is easily maintained, owing to the variety and novelty
of the many different operations carried out in woodworking.
This reduces mental fatigue and ennui to the minimum and
thus prevents any interruption in the continuity of the

treatment. (b) *The attention and concentration* necessary for therapeutic results in craftwork are facilitated by this heightening of interest as well as by the general appeal of all activities embraced under the craft. The degree of attention and concentration in relation to the mental condition under treatment can be regulated by appropriate project selection. This is readily achieved in woodworking because of the wide choice of stimulative or sedative activities available, as well as the extraordinary range in their degrees of complexity. From the simplest activity, such as hand-sanding, the selection moves through every degree of complexity right up to the most complex operation suitable for the most skilled convalescent patient, where less complex projects might tend to develop loss of attention and concentration, so therapeutically undesirable.

(C) *The physical advantages* arise from (a) the *ease in the prevention of fatigue* and (b) the *wide range of joint movements* brought into play.

(a) *Fatigue* is easily maintained under control by the adjustment in arranging light or heavy work to suit individual prescription requirements. It is also lessened by the ease in the prevention of any eye-strain. The gross nature of the working materials, as well as the character of many of the operations, which are of the simpler, non-fatiguing type, call for minimum demand on sight-concentration. The universal interest in woodworking, so easily maintained because of the great variety and consequent novelty of its manifold activities, is a powerful factor in the prevention of fatigue or ennui of any kind. This important feature is one of its main advantages and largely responsible for its high therapeutic rating.

(b) Woodworking possesses a distinct advantage in the occupational treatment of orthopaedic and other surgical conditions, because of its suitability in arranging practically *every type of joint movement* to meet the therapeutic demands of most physical disabilities. There is *flexion* and *extension* of the important joints—finger, wrists, elbow, shoulder, with much more limited movement in the hip and knee joints. In many of the operations there is marked *pronation* and *supination* of the forearms. There is some *adduction* and *abduction*, as well as *circumduction*, but mainly in the shoulder joints. There is a certain amount of *spinal movement*, but this is most marked in the cervical area. Woodworking, owing to the multiplicity of tools, provides marked treatment facilities for disabilities associated with loss of gripping power, arising from finger muscle weakness. While the greater amount of joint movement is confined to the upper extremities, the flexibility of timbercraft activities permits of the arrangement of certain projects, where treatment requirements are confined to the lower extremities. For instance, a treadle-operated fret-saw provides rhythmic alternating flexion and extension of either ankle joint as required, with limited knee flexion—this latter may be accentuated by a sitting posture as against standing. In fact, there is no handicraft which offers such a wide selection of projects and activities to meet the treatment requirements of practically every joint disability.

(D) *The Economic advantages* of woodcraft are based mainly on (a) *the ease in maintaining supplies of materials*, (b) *the relative cheapness in their cost* and (c) *the facility in product-disposal*.

(a) Woodworking is one of the few handicrafts where *continuity in the supply of materials* is rarely interrupted, no matter how seriously conditions are affected, whether by global wars or even local disturbances that may disrupt local commercial interchange. Each country and territory and even intra-territorial regions offer sufficient native and local supplies to ensure an unbroken treatment service. It is true that certain types, including possibly the superior qualities of timber, may not be available in specified centres. This, however, while presenting some restriction of activities, does not create marked interference in the general working of the woodcraft section, because other timbers, indigenous to the area concerned, can be substituted, so as to maintain continuity. In fact, in extreme cases, tree-felling in the hospital estate, where feasible, may create an emergency supply of materials.

(b) The local and native supply sources in timber bear an

*extremely low cost* in relation to the value of a finished wood product or construction job. Even waste or discarded timber pieces or articles can be a very fertile source of supply in most large hospitals and will substantially supplement the local raw supplies mentioned above. Where select woods are called for in any special project, when supplies are available, the raw materials' cost bears a very favourable relation to most other handcraft materials. Even where the cost does appear to be relatively prohibitive, it is more than offset by both the therapeutic and the commercial values of the finished articles. In fact, it is the general experience that sales leave a substantial credit margin and this point is of importance when it is so frequently necessary to influence the lay, non-technical mind in such matters.

(c) *Product-disposal* is a very minor problem in the woodworking section. This is due chiefly to the fact that a very high percentage of the work is covered by hospital replacements or special hospital requirements. This leaves a very small balance of products, the vast majority of which is carried out to special specification, where sales on delivery are guaranteed. Product-disposal, therefore, which may present a serious problem in many crafts, is practically non-existent in all forms of timbercraft and this is an economic advantage which, among the others quoted, helps to give the craft its high rating value.

(E) *General:* Woodworking is a very suitable craft for tubercular conditions as it is possible to grade the work to suit the condition under treatment. Light work is easily arranged in the earlier stages of the treatment and graded up as required.

Whilst a number of operations may be of the individual type, there is some scope for *group therapy* in many of the associated activities connected with the constructional details of many individual products. The preparatory and assembly work entailed in the completion of many woodcraft articles provides group treatment facilities of the easily-arranged type and thus increases the therapeutic value of the craft.

## 7—*Disadvantages*

Woodworking presents many shortcomings that tend to reduce its rating value in relation to willowcraft, basketry and allied activities. These, however, are substantially compensated for by the many advantages listed, not the least of which is the tremendous range of activities associated with woodworking of all kinds, which is not equalled by any other craft, even including willowcraft and canecraft.

(A) The chief *psychological* disadvantage arises from the necessity of restricting treatment to patients who are free from suicidal tendencies and not highly impulsive in conduct. The large number and dangerous nature of the tools concerned call for this precautionary measure. Because of this, woodcraft treatment is contraindicated for quite a number of patients. In addition, there is *increased supervisory responsibility* in the administration of treatment even to patients properly recommended for treatment in this section.

(B) *Physical* disadvantages are of the very minimum and merely refer to the possibility of injury from cutting and various edge tools. Proper supervision and care will reduce this danger, by restricting the use of certain tools to those patients whose mental condition and previous practical experience recommend such a course.

(C) *Technical* objections arise because of the complicated nature of many of the tools and the necessity for some experience in the successful operation of most of them. This difficulty is mainly overcome by the fact that most patients opt for treatment in this section, because of previous skilled or hobby experience. In most other cases, the wide range of the simpler operations in the craft provides suitable treatment and adjustment in the work will keep pace with progress made in each individual case. Where progress tends to show negative or stationary trends, the alert occupational therapist will recommend prescription revision to the appropriate medical officer, who, after consultation, may arrange for transfer to a more suitable centre in such cases.

(D) *Economic disadvantages* may be referred to the large range of tools required and the expensive nature of many of them. While this may have some slight grounds for objection in the initial stages in the organisation of the craft, it can be met by a long-term policy in the system of purchasing where the most essential tools are secured first and thus permit cost of installation to be spread over more than one year. In any case, most mental hospitals, since their very foundation, have been stocked with ample woodworking tools and this discounts the major portion of the objection.

(E) There are some *general disadvantages* restricting the scope of treatment, as compared with other crafts. Chief of these is the difficulty in providing bedside treatment, even on a limited scale. Excluding a mobile treatment unit connected mainly with repair work, the craft is confined to its special centre. Even as a ward occupation, it has an extremely limited application. These objections, however, do not reduce its therapeutic value, as it is capable of giving treatment services to a large percentage of patients, notwithstanding its restriction in regard to locale.

Another general objection is based on its unsuitability for females and seniles. Not many occupations have this dual purpose quality but ample substitutes are available to compensate for this drawback.

In conclusion, a detailed analysis of timbercraft, in all of its many and varied operations, reveals the high nature of its therapeutic rating. The very flexible and adaptable nature of the craft, with the novelty and large range of its manifold activities, together with numerous other qualities and advantages, makes it stand out as a major craft of very high therapeutic value.

# CHAPTER XVII.

## SPECIAL CRAFT ANALYSIS

### WEAVING

WEAVING, as with woodcraft, willowcraft and basketry, is one of the most ancient of handcrafts that are still of popular appeal. Even in the earliest ages of mankind, the original body coverings of skins of animals were replaced by some forms of woven material. There is biblical evidence in Genesis of the use of woven garments of linen and there are records of the weaving of cloth in silk in the Far East, two to three thousand years B.C. Linen weaving is recorded as making its first appearance in ancient Egypt and the large wooden handlooms in general use to-day differ little from the Egyptian counterpart of two or three thousand years ago. It is stated that silk weaving originated in China and the weaving of cottons in India. Apparently, the weaving of woollen fabrics was developed in the colder regions of North and North-West Europe. Weaving from linen and woollen yarns appears in the early historical records of Ireland and Great Britain as well as those of Holland and the Scandinavian countries. Contrary to popular belief, it was not till well into the seventeenth century that the production of cottons on a large scale took place in England and it was only in the early part of the eighteenth century that they became a serious commercial competitor of the older established woollen materials. This change was associated with the application of motive power to looms and this latter development led to the establishment of factory production as distinct from the previous mode of manufacture, which was centred in the weavers' homes, where the hand spinning of the raw fibres was also carried out.

Weaving, whether of the hand or power type, is now a featured occupation, whether therapeutic or commercial, of practically every country in the world. Viewed solely as a therapeutic craft, it varies in accordance with the material used, whether of animal or vegetable fibres, and the type of loom in operation.

Based on the fibres, it may be classified as follows:—

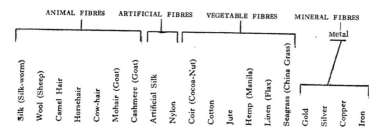

ANIMAL FIBRES    ARTIFICIAL FIBRES    VEGETABLE FIBRES    MINERAL FIBRES

Silk (Silk-worm) | Wool (Sheep) | Camel Hair | Horsehair | Cow-hair | Mohair (Goat) | Cashmere (Goat) | Artificial Silk | Nylon | Coir (Cocoa-Nut) | Cotton | Jute | Hemp (Manila) | Linen (Flax) | Seagrass (China Grass) | Metal | Gold | Silver | Copper | Iron

These cover the vast majority of the materials used in the manufacture of yarns used for weaving of all kinds.

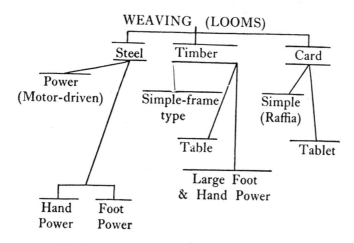

WEAVING (LOOMS)

Steel — Timber — Card

Power (Motor-driven)

Simple-frame type

Simple (Raffia)

Table

Tablet

Large Foot & Hand Power

Hand Power   Foot Power

The above listing covers in a general way the different types of looms used for weaving, but does not embrace specially-designed looms for specific purposes, though these may only be variations of the former. Examples of such looms are *Blanket Looms, Coir-matting Looms, Dobby Looms, Carpet Looms,* etc.

*Weaving* may be described as a method of fabric manufacture by a system of thread or yarn *interlacing*. This distinguishes it from hosiery fabrics where the threads are subjected to a system of *looping* and from lace and net fabrics where the threads are *twisted*. It is also differentiated from felt fabric manufacture, because the latter is a fibre structure as distinct from the thread structure of weaving. In felting, the fibres are pressed into sheets while saturated in a hot soap solution and have therefore no interlacing arrangement of warp and weft threads, which is the basis of true weaving. In the latter, the transverse or dress threads, known as the *weft*, interlace at right angles with the threads running lengthwise, called the *warp*.

Variations in the arrangement of the warp and weft interlacing will create different types of fabrics which are generally classified into four main types.

(1) *Single-made fabrics*, which is the type of general interest in O.T. sections. It consists of only one series of weft threads interlaced with one series of warp threads, (2) *Double fabrics*, where two or more series of threads in either or both directions are used. This gives a strong fabric consisting of either two or three cloths joined together at the edges, (3) *Cross-woven fabrics*, where the warp threads twist round each other, either wholly or partly, interlacing with the weft, first on one side and then on the other side of adjacent warp threads. These are known as *gauze fabrics*, (4) *Pile fabrics*, where the threads are made to project from the ground fabric, forming a pile or plush arrangement on the surface of the cloth. In carpets, velvets and Turkish towelling, the effect is produced by the projection of the warp threads, while in corduroys and velveteens, the milder plush effect is caused by the weft threads.

The special analysis of weaving as an O.T. craft will fall under the following heads: (1) *Qualities* viewed from both the psychological and objective angles, (2) *Economic*, dealing with (A) *Equipment*, (B) *Materials* and (C) *Disposal of Products*, (3) *Technical*, covering all the various operations connected with the craft, (4) *Psychological*, dealing with the mental effects and the nursing requirements in the operation of the craft, (5) *Physical*, dealing with the physical effects concerned in fatigue, strains, etc., (6) *Advantages* and (7) *Disadvantages*.

## 1—*Qualities*

These are considered from (A) the *Psychological* and (B) the *Objective* viewpoints. (A) Weaving, viewed generally, is of the sedative type, because the movements, associated with the action of weaving, are of a repetitive nature. Weaving, however, because of the variety in the many different types of looms and materials used, can arouse stimulative effects by suitable adjustment in the treatment through exchange of looms or materials or both. Apart from the possibility of such changes in the actual weaving, there is some stimulative element present in the pre-weaving operations of warping and beaming, because of the different nature of these activities in relation both to weaving and each other. However, weaving as an O.T. craft is mainly sedative and like willowcraft and canecraft has not the same flexibility as woodcraft in the interchangeability of its sedative and stimulative effects.

(B) *Objective Qualities:* There is a high degree of (a) *adaptability* present in the craft, because of its capacity to supply treatment for practically every grade of patient. This is possible because of the varying degrees in the *range of complexity* associated with the different types of weaving and ancillary activities, providing simple operations and more advanced work as required.

This wide (b) *range of complexity* is an additional special quality of the craft and an essential one for those rated of high therapeutic value. The very simplest type of weave, known as the *plain* or *tabby weave*, is within the competence of most patients recommended for occupational treatment and the work can be made more complicated by the use of more advanced weaves as well as the introduction of colour effects in check designs, etc.

This regulatory feature in weaving creates novelty and a high degree of (c) *Flexibility*. The ease with which change in the operation of the craft is effected makes for the very essential quality of flexibility, which is necessary to maintain its high therapeutic content. Its flexibility is also evident in its application for use in many different forms, not the

least of which is the *absence of restriction* in regard to location.
It can be operated as a bedside operation, as well as in the
wards or at special centres. It is also used therapeutically
for both male and female patients and there is practically
no restriction as to age qualification. Where weaving as such
presents any difficulties for certain types of patients, there
are some incidental operations that may prove more suitable
for such. Examples of these latter are *spool-winding* by
means of hand-operated *bobbin winders* as well as the
insertion of the spools in empty shuttles so as to have the
latter ready for replacement in the *shuttle-box* according
as each shuttle empties off in the actual weaving process.
Another such operation is the hand-changing of the multiple
shuttle-box, when the appropriate colour for the weft requires
to be introduced into the weaving, in accordance with the
design. This latter shuttle-change is automatic in power
looms and in some special O.T. types of looms, but in the
latter should be dispensed with, as the hand changing of
the shuttle provides ancillary occupation for an additional
patient.

(d) *Utility:* Weaving has a most important utilitarian
quality, as practically its entire O.T. output is generally
required for hospital use and this, possibly to a higher extent,
than in any other therapeutic craft. It is possible for the
O.T. department of a mental hospital to provide the entire
hospital needs in blankets, tweeds, towelling, flannels,
bedlinen and general clothing requirements, as well as
matting and carpets of all kinds. To meet all these demands
requires the use of several and many different types of looms
and this gives some idea of the occupational range of this
craft, even if there is a strong utilitarian influence in the
extent of its application.

### 2—*Economic*

The economic considerations are dealt with under three
main heads: (A) *Equipment*, (B) *Materials* and (C) *Disposal
of Products*. (A) *Equipment* is mainly concerned with the
provision of suitable looms, but there is a host of additional
apparatus dealing with the various operations coincidental

with the main activity of weaving proper. These are (a) *spinning*, (b) *warping*, (c) *beaming*, (d) *entering (threading)*, as well as (e) a few *additional accessories* required for actual weaving, the apparatus for these are simple and many of them can be made in the woodcraft section.

(a) *Looms* are of many different kinds, dependent on the product required, as well as on the therapeutic purpose of the work. Such latter would include *table looms*, as well as *bedside* types, apart from the question of complexity adjustment, where very *simple weaving* on frames or plain cards may be called for.

A loom is generally described as an appliance for stretching and holding one set of threads (*warp*) in position, so as to permit interlacing (*weaving*) with cross threads (*weft*). The most primitive arrangement for this purpose was the tying of the warp threads to a suitable low horizontal tree-branch, the stretching (tension) being maintained by attaching a stone to the bottom of each thread. Though this was not described as a loom, it embraces the principles under which every type of loom is constructed from the *plain board* right up to the most intricate *heddle loom*.

It is not possible to give an exhaustive listing of every known type of loom, but the following covers those of general interest, starting with the simplest forms. (1) *Card* and *Board Looms*: These are of rectangular shape and are either matched or holed at regular intervals in the upper and lower ends, so as to allow fixing of the warp threads in position for weaving. These are used for the simplest type of weaving for children or adult patients requiring preliminary tuition. (2) *Simple Wooden Frame Looms:* These are similar to the plain Board type, the latter being replaced by a rectangular framework with a number of different arrangements for attachment of the warp. These latter may be a series of pegs or nails placed at regular intervals on the top and bottom bars of the frame, or merely consist of serrated battens attached to the top and bottom frames. More advanced types of frame looms have *rollers* on which the warp threads are wound, enabling the work to be taken up at intervals as the weaving progresses. *Box-shape frames* are also constructed of a collapsible type for braid or tie weaving with a heddle held in position by some of the warp threads to create the simple shed for the tabby weave. This latter type of loom forms the basis of more elaborate ones. (3) *Box* or *Table Looms:* These give a horizontal warp as distinct from the vertical warp of Frame Looms and allow the use of movable heddles enabling variations in design to be introduced. Because of their nature, they are comparatively small and only produce a narrow cloth, suitable for scarves, belts, ties, etc. They vary in accordance with the number of heddle frames incorporated and the different arrangements for changing the positions of the heddles. These latter may consist of battens at the side of the loom, connected by stringing with the heddles and hand-operated. The heddles may also be connected to a *lifting device* attached to a cross-beam immediately overhead the heddles and operated by strings with wooden-knobbed ends. These strings are held in slotted positions on crossbars, so as to maintain the appropriate heddle in the up or down position as required for the *shed* in use.

Though these table looms may vary in size to produce different widths of braid, etc., they can be made sufficiently large to produce cloths of widths up to 24 inches and even 30 inches. However, weaves of 24 inches' width or greater are produced more satisfactorily on foot-power looms.

(4) *Foot-power Looms* are, in the simpler types, merely table looms of larger proportions set on a stand which enables heddle-changing to be carried out by a system of foot pedals strung to the heddles through a pulley-arrangement on the uppermost framework of the loom. The number of pedals varies from two to six and operate the heddles by means of intervening battens known as 'lams.'

In the less complicated types of looms, weaving is carried out by passing the shuttle from side to side through the appropriate sheds, exclusively by hand. This is a slow process and can be speeded-up, where prescription requirements may call for it, by the attachment of shuttle boxes at each side of the beater or reed frame and where the lower cross-beam of the latter is of sufficient width to form a floor-track for the passage of the shuttle. In these latter modifications, the shuttle movements are effected by manual traction with a strong cord. This method introduces additional upper limb movements to those usually associated with weaving and adds to the therapeutic importance of the craft.

*Foot-power looms*, too, make additional demands on concentration and attention by bringing into play leg and foot movements in *heddle-changing* and thus increase the therapeutic rating value of the craft for both mental and physical disabilities.

(5) *Automatic Looms:* Special handcraft looms, made mainly of steel, have been designed to provide for automatic shuttle changing and shuttle movement by means of either simple leg pedal motions or to and fro manual movements of the *reed frame*, which has a special bar handle for this purpose. This loom is of special therapeutic value in dealing with physical disabilities arising from total upper-limb or lower-limb loss. It has also important psychological values, as it opens up advanced weaving in coloured checks, etc., for patients requiring no special technical skill. It thus can be adjusted for *sedative* or *stimulative* occupation as required. This is possible because of the attachment of a circular box motion, enabling the use of any of six different shuttles to be brought into play, thus creating coloured check and striped designs.

(6) *Power Looms*, being distinct from all handcraft looms, are outside therapeutic consideration and are merely mentioned here as the industrial counterpart of the handcraft types. They, however, incorporate the same principles, whose foundations are laid in the simple frame loom of antique origin.

The automatic loom mentioned in (5) is capable of conversion for power operation, as the hand or leg movements, as the case may be, may be replaced by a pulley-wheel hitch up to any available power supply—such is the smooth and even motion in the hand-operation of this type of loom.

(7) *Miscellaneous Types:* In addition to those listed, there are many other types of looms in use, both of the commercial and handcraft type, that are distinctive because of either

design or function. Among such models are (a) *Carpet Looms*, which also exhibit many varied designs, such as the *Morris type, Brussels type*, etc., (b) *Seaton Looms* for providing a more continuous weft supply and thus obviate the stoppages for shuttle renewals in the plain loom, (c) *American Northrop Looms*, which incorporate an automatic cop-changing arrangement of the shuttle, also to avoid stoppages, (d) *Dobby Looms*, which are used for fancy weaving where the pattern of the cloth requires more shafts than are within tappet control and a special mechanism known as a *Dobby Machine* is attached to the loom for this purpose, (e) *Matting Looms:* These are large steel-framed structures of the very heavy type, suitable for weaving jute and coir yarns and similar heavy yarns into matting to weave floor coverings. They are exceptionally suitable for O.T. departments, as they are purely of the handcraft type and require little or no technical skill in their operation. The shuttle, except in more advanced types, is passed through the appropriate *shed*, from one side to the other, by hand. Possessing heddles, they are capable of weaving check and other fancy designs, by the use of different coloured yarns. The dyeing of these yarns in a special *Dyecraft Section*, opens up an additional important treatment centre.

These cover the majority of the different types of looms that may be found in operation in O.T. centres. There may, however, be many modifications of one or other of the various types described, but they differ only in minor details, as all looms are subject to the general principles of construction, already referred to.

Operations, ancillary to weaving on looms, already related, necessitate additional equipment, as follows:—

(b) *Spinning* is the process of manufacturing weaving yarns, from raw materials, such as wool, flax, jute, etc. Though it is possible to purchase suitable weaving yarns from commercial sources, the fully-developed O.T. department will embrace a special spinning section so as to provide some, if not all, of the yarns required in the weaving sections. Heavy, coarse, woollen yarns can be produced on the well-known traditional *spinning wheel* or on the old type *spindles*.

Such yarns are quite suitable as weft for blanket weaving. The raw wool, however, has to be *scoured* and *carded* and this latter operation is carried out on hand carders, which are easily hand-made. These yarns, so produced, however, have only a very limited use and to enable weaving, as a craft, to be operated as a fully developed treatment service, it is necessary to have finer and better quality yarns available. Some of these latter, however, are capable of O.T. production, by the erection of even a small *spinning installation*, which though hand-operated, is based on the principles of its commercial power counterpart. Such handcraft installations may be purchased from general market sources.

(c) *Warping* is an essential preliminary preparation of fully-finished weaving yarns, prior to *beaming* them on to the *loom-rollers*, in such a manner as to prevent subsequent entangling of the individual warp threads. Warping is carried out on a *Warping Board* or *Warping Frame*, where warps, not exceeding 30 feet in length, are required. These consist of a rectangular board or frame with an arrangement of pegs, around which the warp yarn is wound in such a manner as to secure *figure-of-eight crossings* of the warp at both ends of the yarns so warped. The size of these warping frames is dependent on the length of the warp required. If the latter is of the same length as that of the loom, it can be wound directly on the loom rollers, without previous warping. A frame, 6 feet in length by 1 foot in width, will give a warp of approximately 30 feet long, with a reasonable number of threads. For longer warps, it may be necessary either to increase the length of the frame or by widening the frame, so as to permit the insertion of additional rows of pegs. This warping arrangement may meet practically all O.T. weaving needs, but, if exceedingly long warps are required and particularly where fine silk yarns are concerned, it will be necessary to use a *Warping Mill*.

This *Mill* consists of two sections of framework, attached to each other at right angles and revolving round the central beam, common to both sections. The two sections of framework are also connected at one side by horizontal cross battens, one at the top and one at the bottom, on each side of which are affixed three pegs, around which the *figure-of-eight crosses* are made in the warp threads, as in the warping frame. In this case and also in the case of the *warp frames*, when winding a number of warp threads simultaneously, it is more convenient to feed the yarn by hand from special *spool rack frames*, easily made for the purpose.

(d) *Beaming* of the warp on to the roller of the loom, though a process requiring care, does not necessitate any special equipment, apart from a *raddle* or *vateau*, which is shaped very similar to the reed of the loom itself. It differs in that the upper cross bar, which is permanently fixed in the case of the reed, is removable and is made of wood for this purpose, though the teeth of the comb of the raddle are made of steel or hard brass wire and are arranged uniformly at so many to the inch. Accordingly, a set of differently spaced raddles will be required to suit the number of *portees* (this is the name given to each collection of threads used in each round of the warp on the warping frame).

Beaming is effected through the raddles on to the *cane roller* in the back portion of the loom as distinct from the *breast roller*, on to which the woven cloth is wound on the other or front end of the loom. *Cane sticks* are also used for insertion into the end loops of the warp, the corresponding loop of the figure-of-eight being kept intact by the insertion of a string—each end of which is attached to the corresponding portion of the cane stick.

(e) *Entering* or threading the heddles and reed does not necessitate any special equipment, beyond the heddles, which are supplied as standard with each loom, as well as the reeds. These latter vary according to size required, as well as the number of dents or 'comb teeth' to each inch. The *dents* are simply the spaces between the metal-teeth strips. *Reeds* are so named, because, prior to the eighteenth century, the *combs* (*reeds*) consisted of strips of cane or reed as against the metal teeth since used more or less exclusively.

(f) *Other general Loom accessories* include (1) *Shuttles*, (2) *Bobbins*, (3) *Bobbin Winders*, (4) *Reed and Heddle Hooks* and (5) *Temples*.

(1) *Shuttles* are either of the *roller* or *plain type*. The *roller* shuttles, in use in the larger looms, are of different sizes and shapes to suit the loom shuttle-box and the type of yarn used. The *plain* shuttles may be similar to the roller shuttles in shape and in method of use, but are without wheels or rollers and they may also be of the simple flat type made of bone or timber for simple hand operation, as in the very small *braid looms*.

(2) *Bobbins* are generally cylindrical rods on which yarn is wound for subsequent insertion in the shuttle. Their size and shape depend on the nature of the shuttle used, which is generally made of timber.

(3) *Bobbin Winders* of the O.T. type consist of a revolving steel arm to take a bobbin and operated vertically on the same principle as the woodcraft-type of hand drill described in a previous chapter.

(4) *Reed and Heddle Hooks* are simply timber-handled hooks with an eye, suitable for threading reeds or heddles.

(5) *Temples*, known as *tenter hooks*, consist of a piston-like arrangement, where one narrow square or rectangular piece of strong timber or light steel rectangular rod slides between two parallel arms of similar material housed together at the other end. This latter end is serrated, as is the head of the sliding piston arm at the other end and with a locking device to maintain the serrated ends in a fixed position. It is thus constructed to keep the woven material stretched at a fixed width, so that the subsequent weaving may achieve this uniform width.

(B) *Materials:* The materials for weaving consist of (a) *the raw material* suitable for spinning and (b) *the spun products* into threads or yarns, which are subsequently scoured and dyed into suitable shades.

(a) *The raw materials* consist of fibres derived from four sources: (1) *Animal*, (2) *Vegetable*, (3) *Artificial* and (4) *Mineral*.

(1) *Animal Fibres* are mainly of *wool* derived from the covering of the sheep and *silk* from the silk worm. Other fibres, which are generally not of O.T. interest, are *camel hair* (from the camel), used mainly for hosiery purposes, as,

likewise, *cashmere* from the Tibetan goat, *Cow's hair* used for carpets and coarse rugs, *Mohair* from the Angora goat, used for heavy fabrics and carpets and *Horse hair* for making stiffening cloth for suitings.

(2) *Vegetable Fibres* consist mainly of *cotton* and *flax* (*linen*), which are of most universal use. *Fibres from the cocoanut* have also been spun into ropes and also into lighter yarns for the manufacture of *coir matting* and various types of *coir mats*. *Hemp Fibres* are spun into *manilla yarns*, as are *Jute Fibres* into various thicknesses of *jute yarns*, both, like *coir yarns*, being used for making mats and matting. All these three latter yarns are suitable for O.T. purposes, though the weaving is carried out on a larger and heavier type of steel or steel-timber loom. Another yarn of vegetable origin, derived from the *ramie plant* (nettle fibre), known as *China Grass* (*seagrass*), is a useful O.T. product for seating chairs and stools. *Paper* is also twisted into a suitable yarn for the production of O.T. mats, of a coarse type.

(3) *Artificial Fibres* are also used for weaving purposes. The most common of these is *artificial silk* derived from cellulose or wood pulp. More recently, *plastic fibres* have been manufactured and *nylon products* have also become of commercial importance.

(4) *Mineral Fibres* used for weaving purposes, are mainly of *Gold* and *Silver*, drawn into very fine threads. *Brass*, *Copper* and also *Galvanised Steel* wires are used for grosser weaving purposes. Special machines for manufacturing *diamond-mesh wire fencing* are used in O.T. departments to provide an excellent additional treatment service, particularly as they are procurable from market sources in the hand-operated type. In these, the steel wire is woven into a mesh of varying lengths and widths, as required, though the weaving is not carried out on the warp-weft principle with crossing shuttle, as on the looms described.

(b) *The Spun Yarns*, whether of *wool*, *linen*, *cotton*, *jute*, *coir*, etc., can readily be procured from well-established market sources. They are available in the raw material state or commercially dyed in various coloured shades. Some of the natural yarns so provided may be dyed into different colours, as required, in a special O.T. *Dyecraft centre*, particularly the jute and coir yarns, which do not call for the same technical skill as in the case of woollen, linen and cotton yarns. Such dyecraft centres are a standard feature of most large O.T. departments.

(C) *Disposal of Products:* There is, perhaps, no major craft, where the oft-recurring O.T. problem of product disposal does not present any difficulties, as in weaving of all kinds, particularly in the case of mental hospitals. In these latter, the requirements for finished woven products consume 80% to 90% of the total output from all the various weaving sections in each hospital. The clothing demands in these hospitals are of such a widespread nature as to tax the continuous production efforts of their O.T. departments, and, as a rule, require to be supplemented by purchases from outside commercial sources.

Some of the weaving centres, such as matting and wire fencing, may create a surplus over hospital requirements. There is, however, a ready outside market for the products of such sections, that will cater for a possible surplusage. Hence, disposal of woven O.T. products presents no serious problem in most hospitals and, in this respect, weaving achieves the maximum rating value among O.T. crafts.

# CHAPTER XVIII.

## SPECIAL CRAFT ANALYSIS

### WEAVING (*contd.*)

#### 3—*Technical*

THE VARIOUS OPERATIONS and movements concerned in weaving and associated activities, though of a somewhat technical nature requiring special skilled supervision, are none of them beyond the capability of a wide range of Grade 3 patients. (a) *Spinning* of the simple spinning-wheel kind, (b) *Warping*, (c) *Beaming*, (d) *Entering* and (e) *Weaving Proper*, all of the O.T. type, have been and can be mastered by many patients, in the absence of any previous skilled experience. The actual work must be under the immediate supervision of experienced craft nurses, to prevent serious operational mistakes, or the available consultant technician, when required. It is remarkable the extent of patients' interest in the different incidental operations, as well as in the actual weaving processes and equally remarkable the amount of technical skill attained in these different activities by the patients concerned. The writer has witnessed much proficiency in each of the different classes of weaving projects, covering tweed and blanket weaving, mat weaving and mat-making of all kinds, as well as wire-meshing manufacture, with production results almost rivalling best commercial standards.

It is not feasible to discuss here in technical detail the different operations and movements concerned in weaving-craft and ancillary procedures. A fuller knowledge can only be acquired by having recourse to suitable treatises, which cover the different working details of this universal craft. Many such books are listed in the bibliography given at the end of this Textbook, but it must be borne in mind, as already stressed more than once, that complete knowledge and proficiency can only be adequately achieved in the practical courses covering the craft of weaving. These are a featured part of the training curriculum, whether arranged in the more detailed manner for occupational therapists, or in accordance with the less advanced syllabus requirements laid down for specially trained O.T. nurses. As in the case of the other major crafts, previously dealt with, the various operations, with the many considerations involved, will be explained, with as much detail as theoretical discussion generally allows.

(a) *Spinning:* This is a special type of work, of a nature preliminary to, though not absolutely essential for, O.T. weavingcraft purposes, and the main raw materials, consisting of yarns (spun fibres), can be procured ready for use in the operations preparatory to the actual weaving process.

*Handcraft spinning* of the O.T. type may be carried out on (1) *a special hand-spinning installation,* of commercial manufacture, or (2) by use of the well-known *spinning wheel.*

(1) The special *hand-operated spinning plants,* offered from commercial sources, are of such a bulky nature that their installation for O.T. purposes is generally contra-indicated because of lack of sufficient housing space. They are also not so suitable for producing the finer weaving yarns and this handicap is possibly an additional, if more important, reason for their unsuitability. Hand-spinning of the O.T. type is therefore more generally confined to (2) the use of the *spinning wheel.*

*Spinning* may be described as the conversion of suitable fibres into threads or yarns in such a way as to render them strong enough to withstand the strain of weaving. Though the spinning of flax (linen), cotton and wool may differ in details, the operations generally consist of (1) *cleaning* to extract impurities, (2) *straightening and reducing* the different fibres in parallel fashion and converting them into thick strands, known as *slivers,* (3) *reducing* the *slivers* to *rovings* of the required fineness and then (4) *twisting* the finely reduced fibres (rovings) into the finished yarn.

In the case of wool, which is the most suitable fibre for use on the spinning wheel, the coarse fibre is first washed several times in hot, soapy water (*scoured*) to remove grease and other impurities. It is then carded on a pair of *hand cards* which are short-handled, spade-shaped pieces of hard wood, spiked on one side of the flat rectangular surface with short steel points. A small quantity of *scoured* wool is spread over the steel points of one card, which is held in the left hand, with the points upward and rested flat on the knee when seated for the work. The other card, held in the right hand, is pressed with its points on the wool and drawn in one direction away from the underlying card. It thus tears the fibres asunder while, at the same time, straightening them out and, after a series of similar movements, the fibres, thus straightened, become attached to the right-hand card, which is then scraped down across the edge of the left card. The wool is then transferred to the back of the left-hand card and rolled between the backs of the two cards until the fibres form a small curled roll. These curled rolls are then ready for the actual spinning process, by which they are drawn out and twisted into yarn.

Spinning in ancient times, notably in Egypt and Greece, was carried out by means of a *distaff* and *spindle*, particularly in the case of flax. It is still so used by some primitive tribes. The spinning wheel, however, which is stated to be of the 16th century origin, is of more universal survival and is still a definite active home-craft in most countries.

The spinning wheel apparatus, composed mainly of hardwood, consists of a large, wooden fly-wheel, about 2 feet in diameter, operated by a foot pedal. It has a grooved rim to take a driving band, which is connected to and operates a small grooved pulley wheel (whorl). The latter, because of the relative difference in size with the larger flywheel, revolves at a fairly high speed on its spindle. This is generally a metal rod rotating in two sockets on a special framework fixed towards one end of the top of the three-legeed stool-like structure, which forms the foundation and base of the entire apparatus. Beside the former spindle frame, but towards the other end of the stool top, is affixed a similar though narrower fork-like framework, which, in like manner, houses the spindle of the larger fly-wheel. The foot pedal, which operates the latter, is hinged to one of the crossbars, affixed to the lower parts of the legs for the purpose of strengthening the stool base. The foot pedal has the usual crank-rod connection to the large fly-wheel and is generally made of hardwood.

The former spindle framework is specially constructed to carry out the actual spinning or conversion of the wool into yarn. The curled rolls of wool, as scoured and carded, are fed through a special hole on one upright of the spindle frame and thence along the hooks of a special U-shaped *flier*, on to a bobbin on the spindle, lying immediately between the arms of the *flier*. The latter is attached to the spindle between the bobbin and the socket of the upright through which the carded wool is fed. The wool becomes twisted by the rotation of the spindle and then winds on to the bobbin as the spun yarn.

Special skill is required and attained by steady practice, both in (1) *pedalling the wheel* and (2) on the method of *feeding the wool*. (1) Practice is first required in maintaining a uniform motion of the wheel and in controlling stoppage of the movement when the pedal is just at the highest point of its up and down motion, so as to prevent the wheel reversing, when resuming movement. (2) The actual spinning is preceded by attaching a small run of hand-spun wool, first to the bobbin and then taking it around the hooks on the *flier* and then through a hole on the end of the spindle, adjacent to the base of the *flier* and finally out through an aperture in the upright holding that end of the spindle, to the spinner's hands. To the end of this yarn a quantity of the curled rolls of wool are twisted and everything is then ready for the spinning process.

The wool to be spun is held with the left hand close to the spindle and, when the wheel is fully in motion, some of the fleece is drawn out with the right hand, while the left hand grips loosely, so as to allow the twisted yarn to run towards the bobbin. The to and fro movement of the right hand has to be carried out in a uniform, rhythmical fashion, so as to ensure regularity in the thickness of the spun yarn. This requires a certain amount of skill to get the best results and it is amazing how readily this is achieved by inexperienced patients after constant practice and tuition.

(b) *Warping:* This is a special method of arranging the yarn before it is beamed on to the loom roller and is used for two reasons: first, to prevent the large number of threads, when on the loom rollers, becoming entangled with each other and thus causing breakages and other difficulties in weaving and, secondly, to achieve a fairly uniform tension of the different threads, so as to avoid the loosening of some of the yarns as they move along from the back roller, through the heddles and reed, towards the front roller.

This system of warping is not required for the small box looms, which may or may not possess rollers, as they only produce a short length of woven material. When a cloth, exceeding 2 yards in length and involving 200 or more threads, requires to be woven, as in the case of the larger and wider roller looms, the yarn must first be warped for the reasons just stated. This is carried out on a warping board or frame when the length of the warp does not exceed about 10 yards, as is the case in practically all O.T. weaving centres. Warps in excess of the latter length necessitate a *warping mill.* Both the frame and the mill, as already described, effect the warping on the same *figure-of-eight crosses* principle.

The number of threads required to be warped will depend on the width of the material to be woven, as well as the number of threads used to each inch. Two or more threads may be warped at the same time, as follows: In the case of two threads, these are knotted together at the ends and placed on the first of three pegs, which lie on the top left-hand corner of the frame near each other in a line (the first being about 6 inches from the second and the third a further 12 inches from the latter). Both threads are then carried under the second peg and over the third peg and then around the other pegs placed in a series of lines until they reach the last two pegs (about 12 inches apart) on the top right-hand corner of the frame. The threads pass under the second last peg and over and around the last peg on the frame, returning under this peg to pass this time over the second last peg. The threads are then carried in reverse direction around the pegs on the frame until they reach the original three pegs mentioned above, passing, however, around these pegs in the reverse order of their original directions, that is, under the third peg (which they now meet first) and over the second peg and under and around the first peg. The above process is continued until the total number of threads on the frame reach the number calculated originally on the number to each inch of woven material and the width of the latter.

The principle underlying the operation is the production of the *figure-of-eight crosses*, which keep each set of threads (*portees*) separated from those adjacent to it. To maintain the *crosses* in their respective positions in the warp before removal from the frame, the crosses are tied together by means of a coloured string in three positions: (1) at the crossings between the second and third peg, that is, through the openings made between the crossings and the two pegs concerned, (2) similarly around the crossings between the last and second last peg and (3) the loops made by the first peg are also tied together. The actual method and system of warping is easily demonstrated on the frame and can thus be followed readily by a patient, who, after a very little coaching, easily succeeds in turning out an accurate and faultless warp.

The warp must now be removed in a definite manner, to facilitate its correct beaming on the loom roller. The right hand is passed through the loop made in the warp by the last peg and then all the warp immediately beyond the second last peg is grasped and drawn back through this opening until it makes a fresh loop. The right hand is again passed through the latter opening and the process repeated in this *chain crochet* fashion until the warp is practically all taken up thus. Then three flat sticks, called 'cane' or 'shed sticks,' are used to secure the *crosses* made by the first three pegs. One stick is passed through the loop made by the first peg and the other two sticks replace the coloured string, maintaining the *crosses* made between the second and third pegs. These two latter sticks are tied together through special holes made at each end of the sticks, so as to keep the *crosses* in their respective positions.

The warp, thus removed, is now ready to carry out the

next process of winding on the yarns to the back of *cane roller*, known as (c) *Beaming* or *Turning-on*. The *cane roller* is so called because it possesses a groove on its entire length, into which is inserted the appropriate *shed* or *cane* stick holding the end of the warp, so as to prevent slipping of the yarn on the roller.

(c) *Beaming:* also known as *Turning-on*, is the process of attaching the warp on to the roller of the loom, so that it is spread out and wound tightly and evenly on it. The warp threads have to be spread out on the roller, a little bit wider than the width of the woven cloth. This is effected by means of the *raddle* or *vateau*, as previously described and is available in different sizes, based on the number of teeth to the inch. Where there is a large number of threads (*portees*) used in each round of the warp and also when the yarn is of the stout, heavy type, as for blanket weaving, a raddle will be required which has about 1 tooth to the inch.

The selected raddle is placed at a short distance from the cane roller and the warp is distributed uniformly between the raddle teeth, each portee, when composed of a number of threads, occupying a reed dent. The portee ends are next attached to the cane roller by means of a special canvas attached to the roller, which has appropriately spaced eye-letted perforations for the purpose. The cane roller is then wound by means of a special winding handle, provided for the purpose on most standard looms.

Meanwhile, the yarn is released from its *chain crochet* by one assistant, while another keeps the portees so released at an even tension before passing through the raddle. It is essential to maintain a strong, uniform pull against the winding, as this is an important function of the beaming, to ensure that the yarn, when subsequently unwinding from the cane roller during the weaving process, comes off with a uniform tension and this prevents the development of fluting of the woven cloth because of loose threads. When practically the entire warp, with the exception of a few inches, has been beamed on the cane roller, it is then hold in a fixed position and two shed sticks, some inches longer than the width of the warp, replace the coloured strings maintaining the crosses at the end of the warp. When these shed sticks are placed in position, the winding of the cane roller is resumed until the two sticks reach close to the raddle. The raddle cap is then removed and the raddle taken away to permit the completion of the winding, bringing the sticks right on to the roller. This completes the *Beaming* operation and the next step is to connect the threads to the front roller by the process of (d) *Entering* or *Threading-Up*.

(d) *Entering* is the arrangement of passing the different warp threads through the appropriate *eyes* in the strings of the heddles or *harness* and then through the reed dent of the loom beater and thus on to the canvas of the front or *breast roller*. The latter canvas is perforated similarly to its counterpart on the cane roller.

The method of entering the heddles will depend on the number of the latter and the pattern of the cloth to be woven and it is not possible here to go into detail on the matter, as the work involved must be carried out under the immediate supervision of an occupational therapist or an occupational nurse, who is fully versed in the details and intricacies of the operation. Suffice it to state that the heddles, whether two, four, six or eight in number, which are generally operated by foot pedals or automatically in more advanced looms, move up and down in a fixed manner so as to vary the opening thus made in the warp threads known as the *shed*. This opening or *shed* is made sufficiently big by adjustment of the overall movements of the heddles to allow the shuttle, containing the weft yarn, to pass freely through to the opposite side of the shuttle-race.

When all the warp threads have been entered through the appropriate *eyes* in the heddle strings and proper reed dents in the beater and connected to the front or *breast roller* and the heddles connected up for their proper movement, everything is then ready to commence (e) *Weaving*.

(e) *Weaving* has been defined as:

A process which unites a series of parallel strands or warps by a crossing strand, or weft, which may interlace, wrap or twine as it moves back and forth across the warp strands to form an expanded surface.

The fundamental principle of weaving is the dividing of the entire warp threads into two lines by the movements of the heddles, the upper line containing all the warp threads which require to be above the weft thread and the lower line, those which require to be underneath it. This formation is known as the *shed*, already referred to and the weft is then passed through this shed or opening by means of the shuttle, as it is sent from the shuttle box on one side to that on the other side and the weft thread is then pressed in by the beater.

Weaving, therefore, consists essentially of three operations: (1) *Shedding* or the production of the *shed* or openings, as described. The making of the appropriate shed or opening, to take the weft thread in the weaving process, is effected by the upward and downward motion of the heddles, carrying the warp threads in the *eyes* of its strings. This movement of the heddles is governed by the manner in which they are connected up with the pedals, which operate them. The resultant *shed* following each movement varies according to the latter system of connection as well as the system of *entering* the warp threads, all of which are dependent on the type of weave chosen, described further on. (2) The passing of the weft threads through the shed is known as *Picking*. In many looms, there is a special arm, called a *picker*, on each side, which drives the shuttle, either by hand or automatically, across through the shed. The shuttle is a boat-shaped structure, holding the weft threads wound on a bobbin inserted into the middle of the shuttle, which releases this thread as it travels to and fro across the shed. The cross-beam of the sley, which forms the base for the reed, has the portion in front of the reed surfaced with a *race board* and slightly sloping towards the reed, to form the base of the shed, on which the shuttle *races* across over the lower line of warp threads and under the upper line. (3) The *Pressing-in* of the weft, known as *Beating-up*, which is carried out by the comb of the reed fixed in a heavy beater or *sley*, which has a hinge movement on a spindle placed across the top frame of the loom or, more generally, ⟨ n the lower frame. In the former case, the lower part of the framework of the sley, as against the upper part in the latter case, contains the reed inserted in the groove on the cross-beam.

There are three elementary types of weaves, viz., (1) *The Plain* or *Tabby Weave*, (2) *The Twill Weave* and (3) *The Satin Weave*. These are the three distinctive and simplest weaves on which all other weaves are based.

(1) *The Plain Weave* consists of the alternate interlacing of the warp and weft threads. Each weft thread passes under every second warp thread and over the intervening threads in the reverse order of the adjacent weft threads. When the warp and weft threads are of equal number and thickness the resultant cloth is of a firmer and stronger texture than that of any other ordinary weave, whether a light or heavy fabric is produced in accordance with the relative thickness of the yarns used.

The cloth, thus woven, has a level surface and is devoid of any pattern markings, but a crepe effect can be produced by using exceptionally hard twisted yarns, where the unusual amount of twist develops the well-known crinkled surface, by causing marked shrinkage in the fabric. The special poplin effect is also produced with the plain weave by using very fine warp threads and very coarse weft threads. The former bend compactly around the thick weft threads, giving the ribbed appearance across the width of the cloth. This is usually procured by using a very fine silk warp and a coarse woollen weft.

By reversing the yarns, using a very light weft and a coarse warp, the much heavier ribbing of the *moreen fabric* is produced. Another type of corded or *repp cloth* is based on the plain weave, where fine and coarse threads are used alternately for both the warp and weft. The coarse weft threads cross beneath the coarse warp yarns, the latter being held in a much looser tension than the fine warp yarns, which are held tightly and likewise crossed beneath by the fine weft threads. This creates a much more pronounced transverse rib or cord effect than that of poplin.

The plain weave is of very great O.T. importance, because it is of the very simplest nature and easily explained, even to the most inexperienced patient. In addition, it forms the basis of all simple weaving operations, such as darning, basketry and associated canecraft and willow work, not excluding most forms of mat-making, particularly the coir pile mat, where the individual weft pieces are held compressed together on a warp ground.

(2) *The Twill Weave* differs from the plain weave in that one set of threads is *passed* or *floated* over a set of consecutive threads. This gives a figured appearance of diagonal lines on the cloth, when the *floats* are arranged to run thread by thread in a diagonal direction. When this runs in an upward direction from left to right, it is known as a *twill to the right* and, when running from the right to the left, it is described as a *twill to the left*. The sets of *floated* threads on the cloth surface may be of warp or weft or may consist of *floats* of both sets of threads.

By these variations, as well as variations in the number of threads in each *float*, different figured effects may be produced, which have been given various trade names, such as the *zig-zag twill*, *herring-bone*, *shaded*, *serge*, *Florentine*, etc. In comparison with the plain weave, more pattern can thus be secured in the design, but the woven fabric is not as firm or strong, though a heavier cloth can be produced in the twill design, by increasing either the number or thickness of the threads, in the spaces where the threads 'float' or are not intersected. It must be noted, however, that not more than five threads should be allowed to cross each other without interlacing as, otherwise, the resultant cloth will not be strong enough for normal wear. It is possible, however, to produce many attractive striped, check and tartan designs with the plain weave, even though these be very simple in character, by using different coloured warps and wefts, in a uniform arrangement of the colours.

A *brocade* or *inlay* effect can also be produced by using in addition to the ordinary wefts, subsidiary wefts in bright colours, such as gold, silver, etc., which can be so arranged to produce spots or detached ornamental shapes throughout the woven cloth.

(3) *The Satin (Sateen) Weave* is not, as erroneously believed,

confined exclusively to silk weaving, as it is also used for the production of ornamental fabrics in linen, cotton and wool. The weave, however, is merely a variation of the *twill weave* and referred to as a *broken twill*. Here the direct diagonal line of the twill, using a four heddle harness, is broken by missing the second heddle and arranging it to rise between the fourth and first heddle. This brings the greater portion of the warp to the face of the cloth, with the result that the ribs or lines of the twill do not show, as the weft is almost completely submerged by the warp.

There is a large variety of satin weaves in general use, differing in accordance with the number of heddles in the harness. Satins, therefore, may be woven on any looms with harness containing from four to twenty-four heddles. The *eight-heddle (eight-lam) harness* is the most generally used, as the twill ribs or lines are least visible in this type of satin weave. It can be seen, therefore, that the satin-woven cloth has a preponderance of warp on the front of the cloth and weft on the back. Where the warp and weft are thus of different shades, the warp colour, slightly tinged by that of the weft, will predominate on the front surface and vice versa, the weft colour on the back.

There are other complicated weaves in general use, which require more than one set of harness, such as *double-cloth weaving, figured damask, diaper, plain velvet* (requiring the use of two distinct warps on separate rollers), *figure velvet* (where more than two warps are used). In many complex pattern-weaves requiring special warps as in the latter case, the heddles have been substituted with a narrow perforated board fixed across the loom, which is known as the *draw-loom*. The harness of the draw-loom, which is built in and around the perforated board *(comber-board)*, is known as the *monture*.

All these latter type of weaves, however, requiring special harness and looms are only of academic interest in O.T. weavingcraft. They are referred to here merely to exemplify the many extensions and advances in the handcraft of weaving that have been achieved commercially since Arkwright invented the throstle frame in 1767. Suffice it to say that, notwithstanding the many improvements and additions introduced in the passage of time, the basic principles underlying the weaver's craft remain unaltered, even in the most intricate and elaborate loom machines.

### 4—*Psychological*

As in the case of previous analyses, the psychological consideration may be discussed from the following two viewpoints, viz. (a) *Nursing and Supervisory* and (b) *Mental Processes Concerned*.

(a) The high degree of *adaptability*, so prominent a quality of weaving, opens up its use for treatment purposes to a wide range of patients, covering the three grades, as previously classified. Weaving projects, therefore, from the very simplest card-loom-work, can be made available, both in the wards, even for bedside treatment, as well as at the special weaving centres. *Supervisory responsibilities* can thus be reduced to the minimum by suitable prescription for those cases requiring special supervision. Suitable weaving projects for depressed cases, with known suicidal tendencies, can be arranged at an appropriate treatment centre.

As in Willowcraft and Canecraft, the simpler type of weaving operations on card and small frames can be operated with very little equipment and particularly in the absence of any dangerous tools or implements more usually associated with large loom work, that might, otherwise, have to be contraindicated for many patients. This method of adjustment to deal with supervisory precautions increases the element of *flexibility* and thus the rating value of the craft.

(b) The influence of weavingcraft on the *mental processes* is reflected in (1) *the high degree of interest* aroused. The novelty and diverse nature of the many operations concerned in the craft are responsible for this heightening of interest, which gives the work its characteristic attraction. Although the movements in the actual weaving process, because of their repetitive nature, are mainly of the sedative type, the element of stimulation can be readily introduced by change of loom type, involving greater pattern in the weave, as well as more attractive colour designs. This adjustable feature of the craft helps to maintain the initial interest aroused, which might, otherwise, decline in an atmosphere involving such monotonous repetition, as occurs in plain weaving in one drab colour. The introduction of bright colours in a highly attractive design changes the previous sedative effect into a stimulative one, even on small table looms. (2) *The degree of attention and concentration* called for in weaving is much higher, generally, than in the case of basketry, particularly in the more advanced looms. It can, however, be regulated by project variation, where the simpler work involves much less concentration than the more complex. Even weaving operations of the simple or complex type may necessitate rest intervals to prevent over-concentration, leading to (3) *fatigue*, discussed in the succeeding section.

## 5—*Physical*

The important consideration under this head is that of *fatigue* and its prevention. Fatigue may arise for psychological reasons, where over-concentration may make inordinate demands on attention. This, as stated above, is dealt with by the provision of adequate rest intervals or, where necessary, by the introduction of short relaxation periods and occasional recreational therapy intervals.

Fatigue arising from physical causes may be rectified by (a) *provision of proper working posture* and (b) *avoidance of physical strains* that may be referred to the senses, such as eye-strain or those due to muscular fatigue.

(a) *Working posture* is an important consideration in all forms of occupation, whether commercial or otherwise. It is of particular importance in O.T. procedures to ensure full therapeutic results, as faulty posture may lead to early fatigue and to consequent interference with the general treatment schedule arranged.

In the foot-power looms, a sitting posture is essential, but the standing position is possible with the automatic type of loom, where the weaving is confined solely to the alternate to-and-fro hand-movement of the sley. Where either position tends towards fatigue, it should be possible to effect a change over from one to the other, or introduce relaxation periods with or without recreational therapy intervals, where necessary.

(b) *Fatigue* may also arise from such stresses as eye-strain or muscular exhaustion. Both of these must be watched for and given immediate attention. Eye-strain may be caused by unsatisfactory lighting or intricacy of weaving design, calling for undue concentration, leading to tiredness of vision. Both, in addition, may be aggravated by refraction errors of eyesight. The latter should be corrected before active O.T. is undertaken and the prescription recommendation should give due recognition to the nature of any ophthalmological condition present. Satisfactory lighting conditions should be an essential condition for every form of O.T. project undertaken.

Muscular fatigue can arise from a variety of causes, whether of a subjective or objective nature. The former may be related to the general physical condition of the patient under treatment or to physical disabilities or injuries present in any particular case. Here, both the psychological and physical analyses must have a pertinent bearing on craft selection and the occupational therapist must give careful consideration to the prescription requirements in such cases, to eliminate the possibility of periodic fatigue development.

Objectively, the nature of the weaving operations may create muscular fatigue, because of either over-dosage or project unsuitability. These are avoided by the observance of the general and specific principles and various rules of guidance already enunciated in regard to craft analysis.

## 6—*Advantages*

These will be discussed from the following viewpoints: (A) *Arising from special Qualities*, (B) *Psychological*, (C) *Physical*, (D) *Economic* and (E) *General*.

(A) *Weaving*, as a therapeutic craft, possesses many special qualities, as outlined, which give it a very important rating position among all the major crafts so used. The degree of *Adaptability* and *Flexibility* present as special qualities is exceptionally high, though not equalling that of Woodworking. There is a good deal of variety in the many different types of looms that are available for therapeutic use, as well as the wide range of weave patterns and designs, including colour changes in the latter. This makes for flexibility in use, creating adaptability for all grades of patients. There is also marked flexibility in the complexity range of the many projects available under weavingcraft and ancillary operations.

From the very simple work of plain weaving on cards, there is a gradually mounting scale of complexity in available projects, reaching right up to the most complicated weaving tasks, involving highly intricate colour designs on advanced looms. The adaptability of the craft is further enhanced by its facility for use either for stimulative or sedative purposes, which increases its therapeutic value on psychological grounds.

(B) *Psychological Advantages:* (1) *Supervisory responsibilities* are very much less than those connected with Woodworking and by adjustment in project selection to meet individual requirements, it can be placed practically on a par with Willowcraft and Canecraft in this respect.

Its extensive range of location for therapeutic use, covering ward, bedside and special centres, also enables prescription recommendations to be adjusted to meet any special supervisory requirements that may be called for in any particular cases. Generally speaking, the looms and auxiliary equipment do not embrace any items that might be regarded as of a particularly dangerous nature, as cutting tools are not essential to the craft.

(2) Another psychological advantage, present in weaving, is the *high degree of interest* aroused, because of the variety and novelty of the many operations associated with the craft, as already explained.

(3) Another praiseworthy feature is the *mental satisfaction* engendered in the working and completion of a weaving project, because of easily acquired technical skill even without previous experience. This is achieved after very few trials and without undue supervision and tends to restore the personal confidence, which may have been undermined by the mental condition under treatment.

(C) *Physical Advantages:* The chief advantage on the physical side is the exceptional value of weaving in the promotion of joint movements in the treatment of physical disabilities. Its use as a remedial agent in this respect is enhanced, not alone because of the wide range of joint movements brought into action, but because of the possibility of adapting the various types of looms, so as to secure special emphasis in the case of particular joint movements. This latter adaptation can be achieved for either the leg joints or the arm and hand joints; in the case of the legs and feet by providing special arrangements for the pedal movements and for the arms and hands by varying the position of the beater in relation to the weaver's position.

In this manner, it is possible to provide remedial treatment for practically all the muscles of the upper and lower limbs, covering the various joint movements. These latter include *abduction* and *adduction* of the shoulder joints; *flexion* and *extension* of the elbow joints, as well as *pronation* and *supination* of the forearms; *flexion* and *extension* of the wrist joints; *finger joint movements*, *flexion* and *extension* of the knee joints and movements of the ankle joints.

(D) *Economic* advantages are of a high order in meeting hospital requirements. Weaving products of all kinds, completed in the O.T. sections, find an immediate market in the hospital's demands for these supplies. The saving, so effected, without undermining the primacy of the therapeutic principle concerned, presents strong economic recommendations, which tend to counterbalance the rather high costs of equipment installation and materials.

(E) Some *general* benefits are also associated with the craft. (1) There is ample scope for *group*, as well as *individual therapy*. Each project, with the incidental preparatory operations of spinning, warping, beaming, entering, etc., commands a good deal of team work, which, at the same time, does not hamper the individual nature of many of the craft-work's activities. (2) In addition, the work is eminently suitable for either sex and qualifications with regard to age do not arise with regard to the scope of the treatment. Both young and old find the craft's activities interesting and attractive. Likewise, disease contraindications are of the very minimum. (3) Its wide range of application, in regard

to both mental and physical ailments, is more than equalled
by the facility for treatment extension on grounds of location.
The fact that weaving projects can be made available for
bed cases, whether in the upright or prone position, as well
as wards and special centres, opens up its use in practically
every type of hospital. General Hospitals, Medical and
Surgical, Orthopaedic, Tubercular, Mental, as well as
Convalescent and Children's Hospitals, etc., can all find a
therapeutic use for Weavingcraft in some form or other.

### 7—Disadvantages

In comparison with Willowcraft and Canecraft, the disadvantages associated with weaving as a therapeutic craft
are more marked. These, however, while reducing, to some
extent, the comparative rating value, are not of sufficient
moment to minimise substantially its treatment value as a
major craft. They are, nevertheless, lesser in extent than
those of Woodworking and may be discussed under the following heads: (a) *Psychological,* (b) *Physical,* (c) *Technical,* (d)
*Economic* and (e) *General.* (a) From the *psychological* standpoint, the main disadvantage is the continuous demand
made with regard to attention and concentration. This tends
towards the production of ennui and boredom and consequent
general fatigue. The development of this serious therapeutic
objection may be avoided, as already detailed.

There may, also, have to be some restriction for supervisory
reasons in the case of certain mental conditions, but this
can be overcome by suitable project selection.

(b) Objections on the *physical* side arise from the possible
tendency towards fatigue development. Because of the
repetitive nature of the weaving operations and the amount
of attention and concentration called for in all forms of
weaving, particularly in the advanced types, general mental
and physical fatigue may develop. This, as already indicated,
is counteracted by the introduction of recreational therapy
or rest periods or both and also by proper project adjustment.

(c) There is possibly some disadvantage, on the *technical*
side, because of the very skilled nature of all the operations
concerned in Weavingcraft. This appears plausible in theory,

but, in actual practice, as previously stated, does not present any serious difficulties. The experienced therapist finds that practically all the operations concerned in Weavingcraft fall within the competence of most patients, when this form of treatment is applied by a method of gradation.

(d) *Economic* objections to the craft may be based on the costly nature of the equipment required, as well as the relatively high cost of materials. The latter, too, suffer from marked supply restrictions during war and such emergency conditions. These disadvantages, however, do not present insuperable difficulties and are not of sufficient importance to interfere with rating value.

(e) The chief objection of a *general* nature, is the fact that, in weaving, proper treatment is usually confined to one patient, which appears to be out of proportion to the nature and size of the equipment concerned. This is compensated for through the various associated activities, which provide additional treatment services under each single weaving project.

The bulky nature of the larger and more elaborate looms and, in particular, the blanket handloom, creates difficulties of accommodation, in marked contrast to Willowcraft and, to some extent, to Woodworking.

It will be noted, however, that the disadvantages cited do not offer serious objections to weaving as a therapeutic craft and the fact that it provides treatment facilities, in many different sections of the hospital, enhances its value over all other major crafts. This is clearly borne out by the fact that every O.T. department, worthy of the name, features weaving as one of its most important treatment services.

In conclusion, the principles underlying analysis in general have been detailed and the three major crafts, *Weaving, Woodworking* and *Willowcraft* (*Canecraft*), have been subjected to these general principles. In addition, each of these latter crafts has been analysed in a detailed and special manner, including its history and development. They have been, each, considered from many viewpoints, ranging from the thera- peutic, psychological, physical, technical, to the economic, including the general and special qualities prominent in each craft. The advantages on therapeutic grounds have been discussed, as well as any disadvantages that were of importance. This general and special scrutiny has been covered in such a detailed manner, running through six chapters, that it should facilitate the extension of the analysis to the other major and minor therapeutic crafts.

# BIBLIOGRAPHY

## General

'Office Practice': *William Campbell; Sir Isaac Pitman & Sons, Ltd.*, (1923).

'Lunatic Asylums—Their Organisation and Management': *Charles Mercier, M.B.; Charles Griffin & Co., Ltd., London, England*, (1894).

## Handicraft Therapy

'A Practical Handbook on Leatherwork': *Cécile Francis; Lewis*, (*25th Edition*).

'Artificial Flowers': *R. J. Christopher; Sir Isaac Pitman & Sons, Ltd., London, England.*

'Basketry': *Mabel Roffey; Sir Isaac Pitman & Sons, Ltd., London, England.*

'Bookbinding': *F. R. Smith, F.R.S.A.; Sir Isaac Pitman & Sons, Ltd., London, England.*

'Book Craft for Schools': *A. F. Collins, B.Sc.; The Dryad Press, Leicester, England*, (1934).

'Bricks and Tiles': *Alfred B. Searle; The Technical Press, Ltd., London, England* (*14th Edition*, 1936).

'Cane Work': *Charles Crampton; The Dryad Press, Leicester, England.*

'Cane Work on Simple Frames': *Charles Crampton; The Dryad Press, Leicester, England.*

'Carpets': *Reginald S. Brinton; Sir Isaac Pitman & Sons, Ltd., London, England.*

'Concrete and Reinforced Concrete': *W. Noble Twelvetrees, M.I., Mech.E.; Sir Isaac Pitman & Sons, Ltd., London, England.*

'Design—As Applied to Arts and Crafts': *F. R. Smith, F.R.S.A.; Sir Isaac Pitman & Sons, Ltd., London, England*, (1931).

'Dryad Handicraft Leaflets'—(2 Volumes): *Dryad Press, Leicester, England.*

'Embroidery and Stencilling in Net Fabrics': *Elsie Mochrie; The Dryad Press, Leicester, England.*

'Encyclopaedia of Needlework': *Thérésé de Dillmont; (New Edition in English, revised and enlarged). Editors, Th. de Dillmont, Mulhouse, France.*

'Fine Willow Basketry': *A. G. Knock; The Dryad Press, Leicester, England.*

'Furniture': *H. E. Binstead; Sir Isaac Pitman & Sons, Ltd., London, England.*

'Gilding, Silvering and Bronzing': *Bernard E. Jones; Cassell & Co., Ltd., London, England, (6th Edition, 1934).*

'Glove Making': *I. M. Edwards; Sir Isaac Pitman & Sons, Ltd., London, England.*

'Handcraft Projects': *Frank I. Solar; The Bruce Publishing Co., Milwaukee, U.S.A., (1921-1926).*

'Handicraft for Girls': *Edwin T. Hamilton; Dodd, Mead & Co., New York, U.S.A.*

'Handloom Weaving': *Luther Hooper; Sir Isaac Pitman & Sons, Ltd., London, England.*

'Handloom Weaving'; *P. Orman; Sir Isaac Pitman & Sons, Ltd., London, England.*

'Ink Manufacture': *Sigmund Lehner; Scott, Greenwood & Son, London, England, (1926).*

'Inks': *C. Ainsworth Mitchell, M.A., D.Sc. (Oxon.) F.I.C.; Charles Griffin & Co., Ltd., London, England, (1937).*

'Leatherwork': *F. R. Smith, F.R.S.A.; Sir Isaac Pitman & Sons, Ltd., London, England.*

'Modern Dyeing and Cleaning Practice': *William Brown, M.Sc., A.I.C.; Heywood & Co., Ltd., London, England, (1937).*

'New Leatherwork Decorations': *Elsie Mochrie; The Dryad Press, Leicester, England, (1928).*

'Poker Work': *E. Mochrie & U. R. Fletcher; The Dryad Press, Leicester, England,* (1929).

'Popular Crafts for Boys': *Edwin T. Hamilton; Dodd, Mead & Co., New York, U.S.A.,* (1937).

'Pottery': *C. J. Noke & H. J. Plant; Sir Isaac Pitman & Sons, Ltd., London, England.*

'Pottery in the Making': *Dora Lunn, A.B.C.A.(Design), London; The Dryad Press, Leicester, England* (1931).

'Practical Everyday Chemistry': *H. Bennett, F.A.I.C.; E. & F. N. Spon, Ltd., London, England,* (1937).

'Practical Leatherwork': *F. R. Smith, F.R.S.A.; Sir Isaac Pitman & Sons, Ltd., London, England.*

'Practical Raffia Work': *Edward W. Hobbs; Cassell & Co., Ltd., London, England,* (1932).

'Practical Receipts'—(For the Manufacturer, The Mechanic and for Home use): *Dr. H. R. Berkley & W. M. Walker; E. & F. N. Spon, Ltd., London, England,* (1918).

'Printing': *E. G. Porter; Sir Isaac Pitman & Sons, Ltd., London, England.*

'Recipes'—(For the Colour, Paint, Varnish, Oil, Soap and Drysaltery Trades): *Scott, Greenwood and Son, London, England,* (1926).

'Rug Making': *Dorothy Drage; Sir Isaac Pitman & Sons, Ltd., London, England.*

'Rush Work': *C. Crampton; The Dryad Press, Leicester, England.*

'Rush Work': *Mabel Roffey & Charlotte S. Cross; Sir Isaac Pitman & Sons, Ltd., London, England.*

'Simple Upholstery for Schools and Institutes': *Dorothy M. Hart & John Halliday; The Dryad Press, Leicester, England,* (1931).

'Simple Weaving': *Elsie Mochrie; The Dryad Press, Leicester, England.*

'Soap': *William H. Simmons; Sir Isaac Pitman & Sons, Ltd., London, England.*

'Soft Toy Making': *Ouida Pearse; Sir Isaac Pitman & Sons, Ltd., London, England.*

'The Art of Enamelling on Metal': *W. N. Brown; Scott, Greenwood & Son, London, England,* (1914).

'The Art of Soap Making': *Alexander Watt; The Technical Press, Ltd., London, England,* (1934).

'The Book of Leatherwork': *Mary Woodman; W. Foulsham & Co., Ltd., London, England.*

'The Brushmaker'—(2nd Edition): *William Kiddier; Sir Isaac Pitman & Sons, Ltd., London, England.*

'The Country Woman's Rug Book': *Ann Macbeth; The Dryad Press, Leicester, England,* (1932).

'The Elements of Electro-Plating': *J. T. Sprague; E. & F. N. Spon, Ltd., London, England,* (1914).

'The Utilisation of Waste Products': *Dr. Theodor Koller; Scott, Greenwood & Son, London, England,* (1915).

'The Worsted Industry': *J. Dumbville & S. Kershaw; Sir Isaac Pitman & Sons, Ltd., London, England.*

'Upholstery for Amateurs': *C. Harding; W. Foulsham & Co., Ltd., London, England.*

'Weaving': *W. P. Crankshaw; Sir Isaac Pitman & Sons, Ltd., London, England.*

'Wool—From the Raw Material to the Finished Product': *J. A. Hunter; Sir Isaac Pitman & Sons, Ltd., London, England.*

'Workshop Makeshifts': *H. J. S. Cassal (2nd Edition revised by W. J. May); The Bazaar, Exchange and Mart Office, London, England,* (1922).

### History of Medicine

'Chronologia Medica': *Sir D'Arcy Power, K.B.E., M.B., F.R.C.S.E., and C.J.S. Thompson, M.B.E.; John Bale, Sons and Danielsson, Ltd., London, England,* (1923).

'Dictionary of Psychological Medicine': *D. Hack Tuke, M.D., LL.D. (2 Volumes); J. & A. Churchill, London, England,* (1892).

'History of Medicine': *Fielding H. Garrison, A.B., M.D.; W. B. Saunders Co., Philadelphia, U.S.A.,* (1929).

## Journals

'The American Journal of Occupational Therapy': *Published bimonthly by the Williams and Wilkins Co., Baltimore, U.S.A.*

'The Canadian Journal of Occupational Therapy': *Published quarterly by the Canadian Association of Occupational Therapy, Toronto, Canada.*

'L'Artisan Pratique': *Edited by Rene Leclerc et Cie, Paris, France.*

'Mental Hygiene': *Published by The National Council for Mental Hygiene, London, England.*

## Occupational Therapy

'Craftsmen All': *H. H. Reach; Dryad Press, Leicester, England,* (1926).

'Industries and Occupations for the Mentally Defective': *P. J. Deeley, N.I.H., A.R.S.I.; Birch & Whittington, Epsom, England,* (1944).

'Occupational Therapy': *L. J. Haas; The Bruce Publishing Co., Milwaukee, U.S.A.,* (1925).

'O.T., A New Profession': *Herbert J. Hall, M.D.; The Ramford Press, Concord, U.S.A.,* (1923).

'Occupational Therapy Source Book': *Sidney Licht, M.D.; The Williams & Wilkins Co., Baltimore, U.S.A.,* (1948).

'Occupational Treatment of Mental Illness': *J. I. Russell, M.B., D.P.M.; Balliére, Tindall & Cox, London, England,* (1938).

'Prescribing Occupational Therapy': *William Rush Dunton, Jr.; Charles C. Thomas, Springfield, Illinois, U.S.A.,* (1928).

'Principles of Occupational Therapy': *H. S. Williard, B.A., O.T.R. & C. S. Spackman, B.S., M.S., in Ed., O.T.R.; J. B. Lippincott Co., Philadelphia, U.S.A.,* (1947).

'Psychiatric Occupational Therapy': *G. S. Fidler, O.T.R., and J. W. Fidler, Jr., M.D.; The Macmillan Co., New York, U.S.A.,* (1954).

'The Rehabilitation of the Injured': *John H. C. Colson; Cassell & Co., Ltd., London, England,* (1944).

'Theory of Occupational Therapy': *N. A. Haworth, M.D., D.P.M.; E. M. McDonald, Bailliére, Tindall & Cox, London, England,* (1946).

## Pamphlets

'An Address on Occupational Therapy': *by Richard Eager, M.D., O.B.E.; The Devon Mental Hospital Printing Press,* (1934).

'Memorandum on Occupational Therapy for Mental Patients': *Published by H. M. Stationery Office, London, England, for the Board of Control,* (1933).

'Occupational Therapy': *R.M.P.A., Addendum to the Handbook for Mental Nurses; Bailliére, Tindall & Cox, London, England,* (1938).

'Recreational Therapy in Convalescence and Allied Subnormal Health Conditions': *Frederick Brush, Medical Director, The Burke Foundation, White Plains, New York, U.S.A.; issued through the Sturgis Fund.*

'Reflections on Occupational Therapy in Mental Treatment': *by Corban Assid Corban, M.B., Ch.B., Assistant Med. Officer, Takanui Mental Hospital, Kihikihi, New Zealand.*

'The Revision of the Classification of Mental Disorders': *by the Royal Medico-Psychological Association; Reprinted from the Journal of Mental Science,* (1934).

'What, Why, Where and Who is an Occupational Therapist?': *by Dr. C. C. Burlinghame, Physician-in-Chief, Neuro-Psychiatric Institute and Hospital of the Hartford Retreat, Connecticut, U.S.A.*

## Psychiatry

'Administrative Psychiatry': *William A. Bryan, M.D.; George Allen & Unwin, London, England,* (1937).

'An Enquiry into Prognosis in the Neuroses': *T. A. Ross, M.D., F.R.C.P.; Cambridge University Press, England,* (1936).

'A Handbook of Psychiatry': *John H. Ewen, M.R.C.P., D.P.M.; Bailliére, Tindall & Cox., London, England, (1933).*

'A Treatise on Mental Diseases': *Henry J. Berkley, M.D.; D. Appleton & Co., New York, U.S.A., (1900).*

'Insanity': *G. H. Savage, M.D., F.R.C.P.; Cassell & Co., Ltd., London, England, (1890).*

'Mental Affections of Children'; *W. W. Ireland, M.D.; J. & A. Churchill, London, England, (1898).*

'Mental Diseases': *R. H. Cole, M.D., F.R.C.P., University of London Press; London, England, (3rd. Edit., 1924).*

'Mental Diseases': *T. S. Clouston, M.D., F.R.C.P.E.; J. & A. Churchill, London, England, (1890).*

'Mental Deficiency': *A. F. Tredgold, M.D.; Bailliére, Tindall & Cox, London, England. (1929).*

'Mind and its Disorders': *W. H. B. Stoddart, M.D.; H. K. Lewis & Co., Ltd., London, England, (1921).*

'Modern Clinical Psychiatry': *A. P. Noyes; W. B. Saunders Co., Philadelphia, U.S.A., (1939).*

'Modern Psychology In Practice': *W. L. Neustatter, B.Sc., M.B., M.R.C.P.; J. & A. Churchill, Ltd., London, England, (1937).*

'Psychiatry': *W. A. O'Connor, L.M.S.SA., D.P.M.; John Wright & Sons, Ltd., Bristol, England, (1948).*

'Psycho-Analysis and Social Psychology': *W. A. McDougall, M.B., F.R.S.; Methuen & Co., Ltd., London, England, (1936).*

'Psychological Methods of Healing': *William Brown, D.M., D.Sc., F.R.C.P., University of London Press, Ltd., London, England, (1938).*

'Textbook of Psychiatry': *D. K. Henderson & R. D. Gillespie, Oxford University Press, London, England, (1932).*

'The Invert': *R. H. Thouless, M.A., Ph.D.; The Macmillan Co., Ltd., Toronto, Canada (1928).*

'Twentieth Century Psychiatry': *William A. White, M.D., A.M., Sc.D.; Chapman & Hall, Ltd., London, England, (1936).*

'The Troubled Mind': *C. S. Bluemel, M.A., M.D.; Balliére, Tindall & Cox., London, England, (1938).*

## Psychology

'An Outline of Abnormal Psychology': *W. A. McDougall, M.B., F.R.S.; Methuen & Co., Ltd., London, England, (1933).*

'An Outline of Psychology': *W. A. McDougall, M.B., F.R.S.; Methuen & Co., Ltd., London, England, (1933).*

'Dynamic Psychology': *Dom. T. R. Moore, Ph.D., M.D.; J. B. Lippincott Co., Philadelphia, U.S.A., (1924).*

'Experimental Psychology': *H. Gruender, S.J., Ph.D.; The Bruce Publishing Co., Milwaukee, U.S.A., (1932).*

'General Psychology': *L. F. Miller, D.D.; Joseph F. Wagner, Inc., New York, U.S.A., (1928).*

'Psychology': *E. G. Boring, H. S. Langfield and H. P. Weld; John Wiley & Sons, Incorp., New York, U.S.A., (1935).*

'Psychology': *Michael Maher, S.J.; Longmans, Green & Co., Ltd., London, England, (1930).*

'Modern Discoveries in Medical Psychology': *Clifford Allen, M.D., M.R.C.P., D.P.M.; Macmillan & Co., Ltd., London, England, (1937).*

## Recreational Therapy

'Active Games and Contests': *Bernard S. Mason, Ph.D. and Elmer D. Mitchell, A.M.; A. S. Barnes & Co., Inc., New York, U.S.A. (1937).*

'A Physical Education Workbook': *J. R. Sharman, Ph.D.; A. S. Barnes & Co., New York, (1936).*

'Corrective Physical Education': *J. L. Rathbone, Ph.D.; W. B. Saunders Co., Philadelphia, U.S.A., (1937).*

'Corrective Physical Education for Groups': *C. L. Lowman, M.P., C. Colestock, M.A., and H. Cooper; A. S. Barnes & Co., New York, U.S.A., (1937).*

'Creative Activities in Physical Education': *O. K. Horrigan; A. S. Barnes & Co., New York, U.S.A., (1931).*

'Exercise and its Physiology': *Adrian G. G. Gould, Ph.D., M.D., and Joseph A. Dye, A.B., Ph.D.; A. S. Barnes & Co., Inc., New York, U.S.A.,* (1935).

'Games for Small Lawns': *Sid. G. Hedges; Methuen & Co., Ltd., London, England,* (1933).

'Indoor and Community Games': *Sid. G. Hedges; Methuen & Co., Ltd., London, England,* (3rd. Edit. 1935).

'Indoor Games and Fun': *Sid. G. Hedges; Methuen & Co., Ltd., London, England,* (1934).

'Leisure and Its Use': *Herbert L. May and Dorothy Petgen; A. S. Barnes & Co., New York, U.S.A.,* (1928).

'Leisure and Recreation': *M. H. Neumeyer, Ph.D. and Ester S. Neumeyer, A.M.; A. S. Barnes & Co., New York, U.S.A.* (1936).

'Nervous and Mental Re-education': *Shepherd Ivory Franz; The Macmillan Co., New York, U.S.A.,* (1924).

'Party Games': *Published by W. Foulsham & Co., Ltd., London, England.*

'Play Days': *H. N. Smith and H. L. Coops; A. S. Barnes & Co., New York, U.S.A.,* (1932).

'Principles and Practice of Recreational Therapy': *J. E. Davis, B.A., M.A., with W. R. Dunton, Jr., M.D.; A. S. Barnes & Co., New York, U.S.A.,* (1936).

'Recreation for Girls and Women': *E. Bowers: A. S. Barnes & Co., New York, U.S.A.,* (1934).

'Selected Recreational Sports': *Julia H. Post and Mabel J. Shirley; A. S. Barnes & Co., Ltd., New York, U.S.A.,* (1936).

'Spectatoritis': *J. B. Nash; A. S. Barnes & Co., New York, U.S.A.,* (1937).

'Sports for Recreation': *Edited by Elmer D. Mitchell; A. S. Barnes & Co., New York, U.S.A.,* (1936).

'The Conduct of Physical Activities': *W. P. Bowen, M.A.; A. S. Barnes & Co., New York, U.S.A.,* (1929).

'The Conduct of Physical Education': *M. Lee; A. S. Barnes & Co., New York, U.S.A.,* (1927).

'The Improvised Stage': *Marjorie Somerscales; Sir Isaac Pitman & Sons, Ltd., London, England,* (1932).

'The Philosophy of Athletics': *E. Berry, M.P.E., Ed.D.; A. S. Barnes & Co., New York, U.S.A.,* (1927).

'Textbook of Physical Education': *J. F. Williams, M.D. and W. R. Morrison, M.D.; W. B. Saunders, Co., Philadelphia, U.S.A.,* (1932).

'The Psychology of Play Activities': *H. C. Lehman and P. A. Witty; A. S. Barnes & Co., New York, U.S.A.,* (1927).

'The Teaching of Physical Education': *J. R. Sharman, Ph.D.; A. S. Barnes & Co., New York, U.S.A.,* (1936).

'The Theory of Play': *E. D. Mitchel, A.M. and B. S. Mason, Ph.D.; A. S. Barnes & Co., New York, U.S.A.,* (1937).

# INDEX

U.S.A.:-
History of Development of
O.T. in, 8-9.
UTILITY:-
As Quality, in Weaving, 266.
As Quality, in Willowcraft, etc.,
215-216.
As Quality in Woodcraft, 233.
UTILITY SECTIONS:-
Analysis of, 195, 201-210.
Use for O.T., 66-73.

**V.**

VATEAU:-
In Warping, 282.
VARIETY:-
As Quality in O.T., Analysis of
Willowcraft, etc., 215.
VICES:-
O.T., Analysis of, in Wood-
craft, 243.

**W.**

WALING:-
In O.T., Analysis of Willow-
craft, etc., 220-221.
WALKS:-
As form of R.T., 95-96.
WARD. O.T.:-
Analysis of, 199-200.
Special Room for, 64-65.
Use of Ward duties for, 66.
WARP:-
Definition of, 264.
WARPING:-
Analysis of, in Weaving, 271,
280-282.
WARPING FRAME (Board):-
271, 280-281.
WARPING MILL:- 271, 280.
WASTE MATERIALS CRAFT
Listed with types, 41.
WEAVES:-
Analysis of Complicated Types
of, 287-288.
Analysis of Plain Type of, 285-
286.
Analysis of Satin Type of, 286-
287.
Analysis of Twill Type of, 286.
Types of, 285-288.
WEAVING:-
Accessories for, 272-273.
Description of, 263.
Classification, in Analysis of, 264
Classification of fibres in, 263.
Classification of Looms in, 263.

Definition of, 283.
Double-Type of, (pairing) in
O.T., Analysis of Willow-
craft, etc., 220.
Fundamental Principle of, 284.
History (Brief) of, 262.
Listed, 40.
Special Analysis of, 262-295.
Single Weaving (Randing), in
O.T., Analysis of Willow-
craft, etc., 220.
WEDGES:-
In Woodcraft, 251-252.
WEFT:-
Definition of, 264.
WESTPHALIAN MENTAL
HOSPITAL (Germany):-
Introducing Reil's system of
O.T., 7.
WET AND DIRTY
PATIENTS:-
Treatment for, 33-34, 104-118.
WHITTLING:-
In Woodcraft Analysis, 228,
229, 233.
WILLOWS (Osiers):-
O.T., Analysis of, in Willow-
craft, etc., 218.
WILLOWCRAFT:-
Special O.T., Analysis of, 211-
227.
WIRECRAFT:-
Listed with Types, 41.
Machines for, 121.
WOODCRAFT:-
Analysis of Wood Materials
for, 234-237.
Machines listed for, 121.
O.T., Analysis of, 228-261.
O.T., Classification of, 229.
Timbers listed for, 124-125.
WOOL:-
As Raw Material in Spinning,
270.
Yarns listed for purchasing,
124-126.
WORKMANSHIP IN O.T.:-
Principle as to standard of, 26-27

**Y.**

YARNS:-
Coir, Listed, 124.
Cotton, Linen, Silk, listed, 124.
Spun, listed for Weaving, 274-
275.
Wire, listed, 124.
Woollen listed, 124, 126.